A SIGNET BOOK

DOCTORS WHO KILL

Max Haines was born in Antigonish, Nova Scotia. *Doctors Who Kill* is his fourteenth collection of true crime stories. His earlier work, *The Collected Works of Max Haines*, is considered one of the finest collections of non-fiction crime stories ever produced in Canada.

Crime Flashback is the apt title of Max Haines's newspaper column, which appears twice weekly in *The Toronto Sun*. The column is syndicated across Canada, the U.S., Latin America and Europe, and has been translated into French and Chinese.

A member of Crime Writers of Canada, Mr. Haines resides in Etobicoke, Ont., with his wife Marilyn.

DOCTORS WHO *KILL*

MAX HAINES

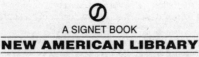

A SIGNET BOOK

NEW AMERICAN LIBRARY

Published in Canada by
Penguin Books Canada Limited, Toronto, Ontario

SIGNET
Published by the Penguin Group
Penguin Books USA Inc., 375 Hudson Street, New York, New York 10014, U.S.A.
Penguin Books Ltd, 27 Wrights Lane, London W8 5TZ, England
Penguin Books Australia Ltd, Ringwood, Victoria, Australia
Penguin Books Canada Ltd, 10 Alcorn Avenue, Toronto, Ontario, Canada M4V 3B2
Penguin Books (NZ) Ltd, 182-190 Wairau Road, Auckland 10, New Zealand

Penguin Books Ltd, Registered Offices:
Harmondsworth, Middlesex, England

First published in Canada by the Toronto Sun Publishing Corporation, 1993

First Printing, 1994
10 9 8 7 6 5 4 3 2 1

⊘ REGISTERED TRADEMARK—MARCA REGISTRADA

Printed in Canada

Canadian Cataloguing in Publication Data

Haines, Max
   Doctors who kill

ISBN 0-451-18393-2

1. Murderers.   2. Physicians.   I. Title.

HV6315.H35 1994   364.1'523'0922   C94-931399-8

To Shirley and Lucille

THE OATH OF HIPPOCRATES

I swear by Apollo, the physician, and Asclepius and Health and All-Heal and all the gods and goddesses that, according to my ability and judgment, I will keep this oath and stipulation:

To reckon him who taught me this art equally dear to me as my parents, to share my substance with him and relieve his necessities if required; to regard his offspring as on the same footing with my own brothers, and to teach them this art if they should wish to learn it, without fee or stipulation, and that by precept, lecture and every other mode of instruction, I will impart a knowledge of the art to my own sons and to those of my teachers, and to disciples bound by a stipulation and oath, according to the law of medicine, but to none others.

I will follow that method of treatment which, according to my ability and judgment, I consider for the benefit of my patients, and abstain from whatever is deleterious and mischievous. I will give no deadly medicine to anyone if asked, nor suggest any such counsel; furthermore, I will not give to a woman an instrument to produce abortion.

With purity and with holiness I will pass my life and practice my art. I will not cut a person who is suffering from a stone, but will leave this to be done by practitioners of this work. Into whatever houses I enter I will go into them for the benefit of the sick and will abstain from every voluntary act of mischief and corruption; and further from the seduction of females or males, bond or free.

Whatever, in connection with my professional practice, or not in connection with it, I may see or hear in the lives of men which ought not to be spoken abroad I will not divulge, as reckoning that all such should be kept secret.

While I continue to keep this oath unviolated may it be granted to me to enjoy life and the practice of the art, respected by all men at all times but should I trespass and violate this oath, may the reverse be my lot.

HIPPOCRATIC OATH
Modern Version

You do solemnly swear, each man by whatever he holds most sacred, that you will be loyal to the profession of medicine and just and generous to its members; that you will lead your lives and practice your art in uprightness and honor; that into whatsoever house you shall enter, it shall be for the good of the sick to the utmost of your power, you holding yourselves far aloof from wrong, from corruption, from the tempting of others to vice; that you will exercise your art solely for the cure of your patients and will give no drug, perform no operation, for a criminal purpose, even if solicited, far less suggest it; that whatsoever you shall see or hear of the lives of men which is not fitting to be spoken, you will keep inviolably secret. These things do you swear.

INTRODUCTION

I am sure that ever since Hippocrates compiled his famous oath, the vast majority of doctors have done their utmost to uphold his fine principles. However, it grieves me to report that the medical profession has had an abundance of members who have strayed from the paths of healing and have plunged headlong into the fine art of murder.

I will not for a moment entertain the thought of placing Dr. Robert Knox in the general category of murderer. Dr. Knox was a well-known surgeon who operated in Edinburgh, Scotland in the 1820s. He also taught anatomy at the University of Edinburgh and required a continuous supply of bodies in order to instruct his students. Nothing was more embarrassing to the good doctor than to face a packed classroom without an obliging corpse lying around.

This imbalance between supply and demand gave rise to the profession of body snatching, a lucrative if somewhat distasteful trade. Two industrious Scotsmen, William Burke and William Hare, didn't have the patience to wait until people died of natural causes. They insisted on giving their acquaintances a little push. It is believed that they gently pushed sixteen friends right onto Dr. Knox's dissecting table. Obviously the doctor looked the other way when suddenly he was being provided with an endless supply of very fresh cadavers. Some say he actually placed orders with Burke and Hare in advance.

When the scandal broke, William Burke was executed. His skeleton remains on display at the University of Edinburgh to this very day. It was only with great reluctance and much urging that a member of the university staff allowed me to view Burke's skeleton. Hare saved his life by informing on his friend.

Although Dr. Knox never stood trial, the scandal ruined his career. He managed to write a book on anatomy and another on fishing in Scottish rivers before he died in 1862. I have excluded Dr. Knox from my personal gallery of medics who have killed because, in the strictest sense of the word and indeed in the eyes of the law, he was not a murderer.

I have also attempted not to fall into the trap of dwelling on English doctors who have hastened the demise of patients, relatives and mere acquaintances, although I must admit the temptation to concentrate on our English brethren was most inviting. There seem to be so many English medics who have diluted powders, plunged needles and otherwise killed for love or money.

In bygone days, when doctors regularly made house calls, many of their patients were lonely women whose husbands had predeceased them. These dear souls grew very fond of their doctors. Some wrote the men of medicine into their wills. It must have been very tempting for doctors with larceny in their hearts to speed them on their way. An added advantage to this type of murder was that the attending physician filled out the death certificate. Between these covers, Dr. Bodkin Adams is a fine example of murder for financial gain.

No book on doctors who kill would be complete without the inclusion of Dr. Hawley Crippen, who buried his wife in the cellar of his home and took off across the Atlantic with the love of his life. Dr. Crippen's crime and his flight from justice provided the ultimate in drama on the high seas. At the time, the world was well aware that a Scotland Yard inspector was following Crippen across the ocean on another ship.

Lest we think our array of doctors were lowlife rounders, I have included the most classic of all medical murders, that of Dr. George Parkman by Dr. John Webster. Imagine such skullduggery taking place within the hallowed confines of Harvard University.

It is distressing to relate that Madame Tussaud's famed wax museum in London has seen fit to take down Dr. Neill Cream's figure. Fortunately, I managed to view the infamous doctor's likeness before it was dismantled. At that time I was told by a member of the museum staff that there was a lack of interest in the doctor. Who would not be interested in this madman, who went around poisoning prostitutes right after Jack the Ripper had performed his nasty work on ladies of the night on the gaslit streets of London? Although Dr. Cream's killing rampage and his execution took place in England, it is my duty to report that Montreal's McGill University ranks Dr. Cream as its most infamous graduate. He definitely deserves to be included in any medical rogues' gallery.

I reached back in history to 1858 to present to you Dr. Billy King of Brighton, Ontario who is representative of all male physicians who fell for the charms of a female other than their wives. Once Dr. King was under the influence of a femme fatale, his dear wife had to go. Dr. King did us the favor of writing a voluminous confession from his cell in Cobourg, Ontario before the end.

These are but a few of the doctors contained herein who, while honour bound to heal the sick, took matters into their own hands and murdered — for love, money or both.

ACKNOWLEDGMENTS

In writing true crime stories, many individuals contribute to the final product.

The various doctors I have consulted in the course of researching material for this effort have requested that they not be thanked by name. They have, however, contributed greatly to my understanding of the different poisons used by doctors who have committed the ultimate crime.

Several police forces in Canada, the U.S., and particularly New Scotland Yard, have been more than generous in providing me with sometimes old and rare portions of trial transcripts which have proven invaluable.

I would also like to thank the staff of Canada Wide Feature Service: Joe Marino, Kevin Tait, Connie Apostoli-Veroni and Nargis Churchill for their untiring assistance and cooperation. Special thanks to the Toronto Sun's Chief Librarian, Julie Kirsch, and her staff: Susan Dugas, Julie Hornby, Bob Johnston, Robert Smith, Glenna Tapscott, Joyce Wagler, Katherine Webb Nelson and Barbara White.

This book would not have been possible without editors Glenn Garnett and Maureen Hudes.

CONTENTS

DR. JAMES BELANY
1843

A few eyebrows were raised when Dr. James Cockburn Belany up and married beautiful Rachel Skelly of Sunderland, England. You see, Dr. Jimmy was 43; Rachel was an unsoiled virgin of 20. The pair wed on February 1, 1843.

Rachel's widowed mother owned several properties, as well as a portfolio chock full of stocks and bonds. Mum was so flush that Dr. Jimmy gave up his practice to devote full time to the administration of her fortune. In fact, the newlyweds moved into Mother's home presumably to live happily ever after.

The doctor and Rachel were married only five months when Mother suddenly took ill. Her son-in-law took care of her medical needs. Dr. Jimmy didn't do that good a job. Mrs. Skelly died a short time after being stricken. Dr. Jimmy stated that the dear soul was carried away by "bilious fever," whatever that is.

Ah, but even the Grim Reaper has his brighter side. All of Mrs. Skelly's worldly goods were left to Rachel. Not one to let grass grow under his feet, Jimmy saw to it that Rachel drew up a will with him as beneficiary.

With the coming of spring, Jimmy planned a trip to Germany to take part in his favorite sport, falconry. He had a bit of a problem. Rachel was somewhat pregnant, but this inconvenience was overcome when it was decided that she would spend some time in London while Jimmy continued on to Germany.

Excitedly, plans were drawn up. On June 3, Jimmy and Rachel rented rooms at a Mrs. Heppingstall's home in

London, England. A Captain Clark and his daughter, who were friends of the doctor, lived close by. It was Jimmy's plan to spend a few days in London with Rachel while she became acquainted with the Captain's daughter, who would act as her companion during his absence.

On the day of her arrival, a Tuesday, Rachel was in fine spirits. She attended the theatre that evening with her husband, Captain Clark and his daughter. Next day, Rachel didn't feel well. She stayed in bed, but the following day, Thursday, was up and about and felt so well she went shopping at 10 in the morning and didn't return home until 5 o'clock.

Later that evening, Dr. Jimmy called on an old friend, a surgeon named Donaghue. Dr. Jimmy explained that he had been taking tiny quantities of prussic acid for medicinal purposes for years and required a small quantity. Next morning, Dr. Donaghue sent a one ounce bottle of the deadly poison to Jimmy's rooms.

Early on Saturday morning the landlady, Mrs. Heppingstall, heard the happy couple moving about in their rooms. Shortly after 7 a.m., Dr. Jimmy requested a tumbler of hot water and a spoon. Mrs. Heppingstall brought them to his rooms. At about 7:30, Dr. Jimmy walked out of his bedroom into an adjoining sitting room and proceeded to write some letters.

Thirty minutes later, Dr. Jimmy screamed for help. Mrs. Heppingstall came on the fly. She found Rachel lying unconscious in bed, frothing at the mouth. Dr. Jimmy was excited, but did not seem to react to the seriousness of the moment. Mrs. Heppingstall hurriedly instructed her maid, Sarah Williams, to fetch Captain Clark. Meanwhile, Rachel went into convulsions. When Mrs. Heppingstall implored Dr. Jimmy to do something, he replied, "It is no fit. It is a disease of the heart from which her mother died some months ago."

Finally Clark arrived, took one look and dashed out,

returning moments later with his own physician, Dr. Garrett. They were too late. Rachel died with her head on Mrs. Heppingstall's shoulder. Dr. Garrett informed the bereaved husband that an inquest and autopsy would be necessary.

The results of the autopsy indicated that Rachel had died from prussic acid, which was found in her stomach. An inquest revealed enough incriminating information to charge Dr. Belany with his wife's murder.

Dr. Jimmy's trial, which began on August 21, 1844, became a celebrated one, chiefly because the jury was asked to weigh a preponderance of circumstantial evidence against one basic possibility.

An array of witnesses was called to the stand and swore that Dr. Jimmy and Rachel had been an ideal couple who had apparently been very much in love. Preliminaries dispensed with, everyone got down to the business at hand.

Sarah Williams, Mrs. Heppingstall's maid, told the court that she had found the prussic acid bottle and a used tumbler on a small table near Rachel's bed. The neck of the bottle was broken. After Rachel's death Sarah had also found broken glass on the steps of the front door, but not in the room where Rachel died. Later the prussic acid bottle was nowhere to be found. Dr. Jimmy stated that he had thrown it away in a vacant field, but it was never recovered.

Dr. Garrett testified that Jimmy had called on him several times after his wife's death inquiring about the cause of death. On one occasion he told Garrett that he had been taking three drops of prussic acid daily for years and had purchased some from Dr. Donaghue before Rachel died.

He went on to explain that on the day of the tragedy he was attempting to take his daily dose when he broke the neck of the prussic acid bottle while taking out the stopper. Some of the acid spilled on the bedroom floor.

3

Trying to be careful with the remainder, he poured it into a tumbler and left the room to write letters. Dr. Jimmy told Garrett, "I heard a scream. I immediately went in a found my wife in convulsions. She said, 'Oh, dear me! I have taken some of the strong drink out of the tumbler. Give me some cold water.'"

It must be pointed out that this statement was given to Garrett before the autopsy revealed that prussic acid had been the cause of death. It is well known that prussic acid gives off a strong smell of bitter almonds. Dr. Garrett stated that he did not smell bitter almonds when he entered Rachel's bedroom. If some had been spilled on the floor, the odor would have been obvious.

There you have it. It was definitely proven that Dr. Jimmy purchased prussic acid, that Rachel drank the prussic acid, and that Jimmy stood to inherit his wife's fortune upon her death.

A guilty verdict appeared certain until the solicitor general instructed the jury: "The question you have to decide is whether the prussic acid had been taken by the wife by mistake or whether the accused had been guilty of the capital offence of administering it to her or purposely placing it in her way in order that she might take it herself."

The jury took only one hour to find the defendant not guilty. However, matters didn't end with the verdict. Dr. Jimmy, who most probably was guilty of murder, was so hated by the public that he was forced to leave London for Sunderland the day of his release. He arrived home in time to witness his effigy being set on fire in front of his house. Three days later, his home was burned to the ground by an angry mob. Dr. James Belany was fortunate to escape with his life. It is reported that he made his way to Newcastle and was never heard of again.

DR. JOHN WEBSTER
1849

The medical profession has an unenviable record in the murky environs where murder abounds. Many a doctor has taken time off from healing and curing to maim and kill.

Dr. John White Webster was a professor of medicine at Harvard University, Cambridge, Mass. He was also the author of several books on the subject of chemistry. The professor had one failing. He tended to live well beyond his means, which isn't that difficult to do if your salary is $1,200 per year. Even in 1849, that was not a princely sum. Besides living high off the hog, the doctor had a wife and three daughters.

To complement his income, Prof. Webster sold tickets to his chemistry lectures. But it really wasn't enough. The professor liked to throw parties and entertain friends just as if he could afford it.

From time to time, Prof. Webster found himself in such dire financial straits that he was forced to borrow money from an affluent colleague, Dr. George Parkman. Dr. Parkman had loaned Webster $400 some seven years earlier. The loan was secured by a promissory note and a mortgage on some of the professor's personal property.

When Prof. Webster had difficulty paying off the note, Dr. Parkman came to his aid once again. The doctor, with some other men, loaned the professor a further $2,432. This loan was secured by a mortgage on all of Webster's personal property, including a valuable mineral collection.

Nothing seemed to alleviate Webster's financial woes.

He approached Dr. Parkman's brother-in-law, Robert Shaw, gave him a hard-luck story and succeeded in selling him his mineral collection for $1,200. By chance, Parkman and Shaw were discussing Webster and his tight financial situation when the subject of the mineral collection came up. Dr. Parkman was furious to find out that Webster had sold an item on which he held the mortgage. In the weeks that followed, Dr. Parkman put real heat on Webster, threatening legal action if the professor failed to ante up.

On a Friday in November 1849, Dr. Parkman had an appointment to meet Prof. Webster in his laboratory. Dr. Parkman arrived at 1:45 p.m. No one could remember ever seeing him again.

Two days after Dr. Parkman disappeared, Prof. Webster paid a visit to his colleague's brother's home. Rev. Parkman was somewhat surprised to see Webster. The professor told the minister that he had met with Dr. Parkman the previous Friday and had paid him $483 against the money he owed. He said that the doctor had rushed out of his laboratory and apparently no one had seen him since that time.

A man of Dr. Parkman's stature doesn't go missing every day. His disappearance was the talk of the university campus, if not all of Boston. By paying a visit to the missing man's brother , Prof. Webster lent credence to those who believed that the doctor had been attacked, robbed and quite possibly murdered. It was these rumors which came to the attention of a man named Littlefield, who was the janitor of the building housing Prof. Webster's laboratory.

Littlefield decided to make a thorough search of the premises. He had found it strange that the professor had double locked his vault-like laboratory, which was situated below his living quarters. The lab contained a huge furnace.

Using a crowbar, Littlefield worked at breaking through the wall of the lab. His wife stood guard in case Webster showed up. It was slow going, taking the better part of a night. Finally, he broke through and poked his torch inside. "I held my light forward and the first thing which I saw was the pelvis of a man and two parts of a leg. The water was running down on these remains from the sink. I knew it was no place for these things."

University officials and the police were notified. Dr. Webster was taken into custody. Here was a distinguished man of letters incarcerated for taking the life of an equally distinguished colleague. Dr. Webster was a Master of Arts, a medical doctor, a member of the American Academy of Arts and Sciences. The list was as long as your arm. In custody, he was near collapse.

Dr. Webster's trial captured headlines throughout North America. To facilitate the thousands who wished to attend, the courtroom was cleared every 15 minutes so that a new group of spectators could gain entrance. In this way, thousands could later claim they had attended the famous murder trial of Prof. Webster. The trial itself lasted 11 days.

Janitor Littlefield was one of the main witnesses for the prosecution. He explained that Dr. Webster's lab was more of a vault where body parts were delivered from the dissecting room. They were burned in Webster's furnace. On the evening of Dr. Parkman's disappearance, Littlefield had seen him walking towards Webster's flat, but had not seen him enter.

During the next few days, while scores of officials were searching for the missing Dr. Parkman, the professor had locked himself in his vault for hours on end. Fires were kept burning in the furnace and water could be heard steadily running in the vault. The vault gave up several human body parts and fragments of teeth were found in the furnace.

Defence counsel attempted to raise doubts over the body parts, claiming that they were not those of the good doctor. It was further claimed that even if the human remains were those of Dr. Parkman, it was quite possible that someone else had placed the parts in the vault to incriminate Prof. Webster. Defence counsel even suggested that Littlefield himself had as much opportunity to do away with the doctor as did Webster.

In the end, the trial hinged on whether or not the body parts were indeed Dr. Parkman's mortal remains. This was proven without a doubt when false teeth found in the furnace were produced in evidence. Dr. Nathan Keep, a friend of both Parkman and Webster, had retained the molds he had made when fitting Dr. Parkman's teeth. The teeth found in the furnace fit the molds exactly. Dr. Keep cried as he gave evidence, fully aware that he was sealing the fate of a good friend.

The evidence, totally circumstantial, for no one had seen the two men together, was now in. The jury retired for only three hours before returning with a verdict of guilty.

Prof. Webster was given the opportunity to make a statement. Following is a pertinent portion of that statement: "Repeating in the most solemn and positive manner, and under the fullest sense of my responsibility as a man and as a Christian, that I am wholly innocent of this charge, to the truth of which the Searcher of all hearts is a witness."

The statement was heart rending and caused many a tear to flow. It was a pack of lies.

Some weeks later, Webster withdrew his courtroom statement and wrote out a detailed confession. He told how Parkman had approached him in a gruff manner demanding, "Have you got the money?" Webster replied, "No, doctor." He went on to state that he had attempted to explain his position but was constantly interrupted and called a liar and a scoundrel. When Parkman waved mortgage papers in his face, he couldn't control himself. He picked up the closest weapon at hand, a piece of wood, and brought in down full force on Parkman's head. The doctor didn't move. He was dead.

According to his own statement, Webster never gave a thought to calling for assistance. He immediately thought of disposing of the body to avoid being suspected. Webster dragged the body into an adjacent room and removed the doctor's clothing and the contents of his pockets. Both were burned in the furnace. The body was dismembered in the sink while the water kept running, moving blood down the drain.

Prof. Webster pleaded for his life, claiming that he had acted in a fit of anger. He also apologized to Littlefield for having his lawyer cast suspicion in the janitor's direction. His confession did nothing to save his life, but it did provide us with certain insights. Respectable professional men who have never committed a violent act in their lives are capable of murder. They can also lie eloquently from the witness stand.

Dr. John White Webster was hanged for the murder of Dr. George Parkman on the last Friday in August 1850.

DR. WILLIAM PALMER
1855

Poisoners as a group have always plied their dubious profession under an extreme disadvantage. They simply have to obtain their poison somewhere. Invariably a chemist or pharmacist ends up on the witness stand pointing a finger at the accused exclaiming, "He said it was to get rid of rats," or some other innocuous expression designed to lend legitimacy to the purchase.

That is, unless the accused happens to be a *doctor*.

Dr. William Palmer was born on October 21, 1824 in Rugeley, England and took his medical degree in London. During his student days he gained quite a reputation as a gambler with a particular affinity for the ponies. He returned to Rugeley and married a colonel's daughter, Annie Brooks. Everything went along well with the doctor and his wife as he established a large and profitable practice. Dr. Palmer neither smoked nor drank, and who are we to criticize if he bet a bob or two on the horses now and then. The Palmers lived in a big house, and he appeared to have everything any man could want.

Then one day an annoying lady from Rugeley presented him with an illegitimate child. Being a man of medicine he thought it would be a good idea to give the newborn child a physical examination. The child died of convulsions shortly after the visit to the doctor's office.

Dr. Palmer and Annie proceeded to have five children during the course of their marriage, and all but one died of convulsions. The eldest, Willie, through the luck of the draw, outlived dear old Dad.

After the initial pleasures of married life had worn off,

Dr. Palmer started to bet heavily on the horses. Then, as now, it was very difficult to beat the nags and he got deeper and deeper into debt. Finally his mother-in-law, Mrs. Thornton, was approached for a loan. She sent him 20 pounds, and in effect told him to get lost. William, never one to pass up a mark, invited Mrs. Thornton to come stay with him and Annie. She was dead within two weeks, and the Palmers inherited nine houses. The doctor was furious when he found out they were in need of repair.

Then Dr. Palmer invited an acquaintance of his, Mr. Bladon, to visit. He owed Bladon several hundred pounds, which he promised to pay back during his stay. Poor Bladon was hardly settled in the house before he passed away suddenly during the night, writhing with convulsions. Dr. Palmer was obviously distressed at losing his friend. He brought in a colleague, Dr. Bamford, during that last horrible night, and it was Dr. Bamford who signed the death certificate with the cause of death being English cholera. In all fairness, we should point out that 80-year-old Dr. Bamford was a tottering, half-blind gentleman who looked up to Dr. Palmer and was flattered at being consulted. Kindly Dr. Palmer took care of his friend's funeral arrangements. He was even decent enough to tell Bladon's widow that while her husband owed him huge sums of money, under the circumstances, he would forget the debt.

Another gentleman named Bly was hounding Palmer for £800 when he was invited down to Rugeley for a visit. Exit Bly.

Around now, Mrs. Palmer was beginning to wonder. First her children, and now it seemed that everyone who walked into their front door was being carried out. She didn't have all that long to worry. Mrs. Palmer attended a concert in Liverpool on the night of September 18, 1854 and took a slight chill. Dr. Palmer prescribed bed rest.

Their servant, Eliza Thorn, was preparing Mrs. Palmer's meals, but the considerate doctor insisted on carrying them upstairs and feeding his wife. The patient vomited continuously and grew weaker. Dr. Bamford was called in and was told by Dr. Palmer that his wife had English cholera. She was dead in two weeks. Dr. Bamford duly signed the death certificate, and Palmer collected £13,000 in insurance money.

By now William had his own string of horses, and the added expense of trainers, stables and jockeys. His horses can best be described as slow. The doctor was spending money faster than he could kill people.

William, who never drank himself, had a brother who was an alcoholic. He convinced his brother that he would give him a loan which the brother would never have to pay back. William would take out insurance on his life, and when he died Dr. Palmer would get his money back. The brother, Walter, who was in a daze most of the time, went for it. Dr. Palmer sobered him up long enough to pass the physical exam required by the insurance company. You guessed it. Walter passed away, and Dr. Palmer again collected £13,000 insurance.

Still the flow of money coming in wasn't enough, and soon Dr. Palmer was borrowing from loan sharks and paying 60 per cent interest. The money lender, Mr. Pratt, demanded money on certain dates, and unlike previous lenders, he would not be put off.

One day at the race track, Dr. Palmer met John Parsons Cook. Now Cook was a friend cut from the same cloth as Palmer. He had his own stable and was a hard-drinking playboy. One day at the races Cook had a long shot come in by a nose. The men had a champagne supper and some further drinks to celebrate. During the celebration Palmer gave Cook some brandy, and he immediately took ill. When it came time to return to Rugeley, Palmer suggested that Cook return with him.

There were comfortable lodgings at the Talbot Arms, right across the street from his own house. Cook thought the doctor most obliging, and the two men left together.

Once installed at the Talbot Arms, Cook's illness became worse. The more Dr. Palmer prescribed for him, the worse he became. Finally he died. After he passed away, Palmer produced cheques in his favor signed by Cook. The doctor was making his usual hasty funeral arrangements for his friend, when a spoilsport arrived on the scene. Cook's stepfather, a Mr. Stevens, advised Palmer that he would make all the arrangements. In fact, he thought the whole thing smelled to high heaven. Stevens was going to have a post mortem performed on Cook's body and an inquiry into his death.

On Friday, December 14, the results of the post mortem were presented at the inquiry. No strychnine was found in the body, but the cause of death was given as tetanus which was the result of the administration of strychnine. A verdict of wilful murder was returned against Dr. Palmer.

The whole of England talked of little else but the Dr. William Palmer case. There were many who couldn't believe that the gambler and mass murderer described by the newspapers was the same gentle doctor they knew. The bodies of his wife Annie and his brother Walter were exhumed. Annie's body was found to contain antimony. While no poison was evident in Walter's body, it was believed that he met his death by the administration of prussic acid. Traces of this acid would have evaporated since death.

Dr. Palmer's house and the Talbot Arms became so notorious that an enterprising photographer set up his equipment in front of the two establishments. For a small sum you could have your picture taken with the murder buildings in the background. Dr. Palmer was speedily found guilty of murder. In 1855, there were still public executions in England. Before a howling crowd, shouting "Poisoner, poisoner!" Dr. Palmer was hanged. He was 31 years old.

DR. WILLIAM KING
1858

Today, the town of Brighton, Ontario is off the beaten path. Located about 100 miles east of Toronto, only a green sign on a superhighway indicates the exit to the peaceful little town.

Years ago, before the Macdonald-Cartier Freeway was built between Toronto and Montreal, Canada's two largest cities, it was necessary to travel through Brighton. In horse and buggy days the town was a main stopover. It was here, back in 1858, that murder so very foul took place, a murder which would capture the attention of the entire country.

William Henry King was born in 1833 on a farm just outside Brighton in the township of Sophiasburg. His parents moved to Brighton, where young William spent his formative years. At the age of five, he was sent off to school, where he displayed a remarkable aptitude to learn and absorb. We must remember that we are delving back into a time when schooling was not always available, even to those who were recognized as gifted children. William's main activity as he grew up was helping out on the farm which, in a few short years, became relatively prosperous.

The young man with the driving ambition was pleasant and charming. He stood five feet eleven inches tall and sported a lush growth of sandy whiskers, which was in keeping with the style of the times.

At the age of 18, William attended normal school in Toronto. Each summer he returned home to work on the family farm. During one of these summers, he started to date Sarah Ann Lawson. Ann, as she was known, left quite a bit to be desired in the looks department. She wore a perpetual frown, which gave her a rather stern appearance. Her personality was diametrically opposite to what one would describe as warm.

The powers that be have a way of evening things out. Ann's father was loaded. John M. Lawson owned a large, prosperous farm and was widely respected throughout the area. Can't you just hear the ladies of Brighton gossiping in the general store over a bolt of gingham — "That handsome King boy is after the Lawson money."

On January 31, 1855, William and Ann were married. While he continued his studies, his dutiful wife took in boarders to help defray the cost of his education. In Toronto, William obtained a first class teacher's certificate. He returned to Brighton, where he taught for a few months before obtaining a position as a third class teacher at Hamilton Central School.

About a year after their marriage, Ann gave birth to a daughter, who was sickly from the day she was born. The child lived for only a little more than a month. It was around this time that a rather ugly rumor circulated about the King marriage. The good folks of Brighton whispered that William mistreated his wife. The rumors were given some credence when Ann did what so many other women have done before and since. She went home to mother.

William's driving ambition would not be stifled. He threw himself into a new career, that of medicine. With his father- in- law's financial assistance, he enrolled in Philadelphia's Hom-eopathy Medical College. Meanwhile, Ann remained under her parents' roof in Brighton. William stayed in Philadelphia for three years, returning home each summer to teach in local schools between college semesters. During one semester, he wrote his wife several letters accusing her of infidelity, a totally bogus accusation. Anne showed the letters to her father, who was so upset he took them to his lawyer. When William apologized, his father-in-law agreed to return the letters. The wily Mr. Lawson took the precaution of copying the strange missives.

In 1858, William King returned to his home town. He was now a bona fide doctor, having graduated from the Homeopathy Medical College, Pennsylvania Medical University and the Eclectic Medical College.

Dr. King hung out his shingle. Right from the beginning, his practice prospered. And why not? Here was a local boy who had displayed the fortitude and determination to better himself. Besides, William dressed well, was always nicely groomed and had a delightful bedside manner. He and Ann reconciled. Everything was coming up roses, until that fall of 1858. Actually, it was exactly September 23 when the bloom came off the rose and love flew out the window, for on that day William King first laid eyes on Melinda Freeland Vandervoort.

It wasn't that the good doctor had eyes only for Melinda. Nothing could be further from the truth. He had simultaneously made advances to a patient, Dorcas Garrett, of nearby Murray. That was a mistake. Dorcas, a Quaker, was just not that type of woman. William had sent her a letter expressing undying love. He insinuated that his dear wife was not long for this world and added that Dorcas should acquaint herself with the niceties of life befitting a doctor's wife.

As I said, Dorcas wasn't having any. She replied in no uncertain terms that she was dismissing him as her physician and at the same time demanded an apology. She threatened to expose him if he made any further advances. William apologized.

Melinda was another kettle of fish. She responded to the doctor's letter by sending him a photograph with an accompanying letter containing such titillating lines as "You have unlinked the tender chord of affection until you have an alarming influence over my girlish nature," and, "One smile from your countenance can inspire a depth of veneration in my bosom never felt by me for any individual."

William had struck paydirt. The pair corresponded. It didn't matter one iota that Ann King was two months pregnant. Her husband wrote Melinda that she was very ill and could die at any moment. If Melinda would just wait for another year, she would become the second Mrs. King. When these letters were written, Ann was in perfect health.

Four days after William wrote Melinda concerning his wife's condition, Ann took ill. She vomited continuously, suffered excruciating pains in her stomach and complained of a burning sensation in her throat. During the initial stages of his wife's illness, William provided her sole medical care. He told Ann's family that she was suffering from ulcerations of the womb and that everything possible was being done. So concerned was William that he rarely left his wife's bedside. For three weeks, William labored over his patient. Some days she seemed to rally, but always slipped back into bouts of vomiting and retching. During the few times Ann was lucid, she implored her husband to stop giving her that hideous white powder five times a day. She complained that it "burned like fire" in her mouth.

Finally, as Ann grew weaker, William succumbed to Mr. Lawson's urging and sought a second medical opinion. Dr. A. E. Fife was told by William that the patient was pregnant and had ulcerations of the womb. The doctor was not asked, nor did he request, to examine Ann. He prescribed ipecacuanha and camphor to alleviate the vomiting.

Nothing seemed to help Ann King. Once again, Mr. Lawson begged his son-in-law to bring in additional medical assistance. Dr. P. Gross was given the same information as Dr. Fife. He too prescribed something to help stem the insistent vomiting.

Who knows what thoughts raced through Ann's mind as she lay there in agony? Certainly she was aware that her husband was carrying on with the rather notorious 20-year-old Melinda Vandervoort. No doubt word drifted back to her of her husband's house calls to rural areas with the ever present Melinda at his side. Sometimes, Melinda actually cared for Ann in the doctor's absence.

On November 4, 1858, Ann died. Dr. King was beside himself with grief. In fact, he carried on so much that witnesses were in fear for his life. The man convulsed, grew crimson in the face and required medical assistance.

Ann's parents never did like their son-in-law. Now that the worst had happened, they decided to find out once and for all if their suspicions were based on fact. While William was out of the house, Mrs. Lawson searched the premises. She came up with a photo of Melinda Vandervoort, along with incriminating letters from Melinda written to William insinuating how convenient it would be to have Ann out of the way.

On Sunday, November 7, Ann was buried. Dr. King was disconsolate. The following day, Ann's brother Clinton went to the county coroner with an array of incriminating evidence. He lugged along the accusatory letters his father had copied, as well as letters from Melinda to William and the letter written by William to Dorcas Garrett. As soon as she had heard of Ann's death, Dorcas had turned it over to Ann's brother.

The Lawsons demanded an inquest into their daughter's death and informed William that an autopsy was to be performed. He was furious, but not so distraught that he didn't proceed directly to Sidney and the everloving arms of Melinda Vandervoort.

Once the ball started to roll, there was no stopping it. A coroner's jury was hastily convened and Ann's body exhumed. An autopsy revealed that there was no ulceration of the womb. The stomach and its contents were removed for analysis.

Meanwhile William, no doubt realizing what the autopsy would reveal, had a meeting with Melinda at her home in Sidney. While at the Vandervoorts, William met Melinda's father for the first time. He told both father and daughter that he and Melinda were in trouble due to his wife's death. He would be arrested and so would Melinda. He implored Mr. Vandervoort for permission to flee with Melinda to Cape Vincent in New York state, where Melinda's aunt lived. William was lying, as he wasn't being sought by the law just yet, but the ploy worked. Mr. Vandervoort allowed his daughter to flee with Dr. King.

A warrant was soon issued for William's arrest. He was apprehended, brought back to Canada, charged with murder and lodged in jail. Melinda, who had made her way to Cleveland, Ohio, returned to Brighton three weeks later. On April 4, 1859, Dr. William King stood trial for the murder of his wife. Farmers travelled to the trial by horse and buggy. Those who couldn't get a lift walked to the tiny Cobourg courthouse where the trial was held. It was estimated that 1500 people attempted to attend the proceedings, but only a fraction of that number gained admittance. King gave the appearance of tolerating the entire distasteful affair.

The Crown went about building its formidable case. The accused man had opportunity and motive. He had predicted his wife's death while she was still in good health and had invented a nonexistent illness to ward off other doctors and to account for her death. Professor Henry Croft of Toronto's University College testified that he had examined the deceased's stomach. It was found to contain 11 grains of arsenic. The liver contained small quantities of arsenic as well. This was vital evidence, as explained by Prof. Croft from the witness stand: "Arsenic cannot be put into the liver after death." Defence counsel's main thrust was that arsenic could have been placed in the stomach after death.

Ann's mother took the witness stand and tearfully related that she had watched William mix a white powder with water and administer it to her daughter. Most of the time Ann vomited and retched after each dose. She did admit under cross-examination that, on occasion, Ann's condition had appeared to improve slightly.

Melinda Vandervoort was called to testify. She accounted for her involvement with Dr. King with a few well chosen answers. In response to what everyone was thinking, she replied, "I never had any improper intercourse with Dr. King." Melinda gave the following explanation for replying to suggestive letters she had received from the doctor, as well as sending him her photograph. Melinda said, "Mrs. King asked me to send the likeness to her. I directed the likeness to Dr. King. I thought that when I got the letter, it was written for amusement. I sent him this letter in answer for amusement."

No one really believed Melinda. After receiving Melinda's photograph, William dashed off a reply to his "Sweet little lump of good nature." In part, he wrote, "Could I indulge in the hope that those winning and genial smiles would ever be found in my possession, all troubles would then cease. It is a perfect infatuation to me. Can you keep from sacrificing yourself upon the hymeneal altar for the next year? I wish so."

Melinda responded with such tasty tidbits as, "Since I first had the pleasure of an introduction, my heart is constantly with you, and I'm not contented a moment. O could I forever be with you; I think I should be happy, for indeed I enjoyed myself to excess during my stay in your presence though suppose now I must eradicate such thoughts from my mind; for you are married, and my destiny must be to love and not share your interesting society."

The defence paraded an impressive array of doctors who testified to Dr. King's high moral standards, as well as his medical knowledge and skill. The defence made much of the fact that there was opportunity for arsenic to have been placed in the stomach contents after death. This was vehemently refuted by the Crown.

The jury retired to deliberate their verdict. When they had difficulty reaching a decision in a few hours, they were sequestered overnight. Promptly at 10 a.m., before a crowded but dead silent courtroom, the clerk of the court asked the question on everyone's mind, "How say you gentlemen, is the prisoner guilty or not guilty?" The foreman of the jury replied, "Guilty, with a strong recommendation to mercy."

On Saturday, April 9, Dr. King was once again led into the Cobourg courtroom for sentencing. When asked if he had anything to say before being sentenced, he replied, "I have this much to say, that upon my solemn oath I am not guilty of the charge laid against me. I have no doubt of this; my conscience is perfectly clear upon this point." The presiding judge then sentenced King to be hanged on June 9, 1859. Dr. King wept as he was led away to await his date with the hangman.

While in prison, William confessed to his spiritual advisor, Rev. Vanderburg, that he was guilty of having murdered his wife. Then, quite unlike most killers, he wrote out his confession in detail. Following are excerpts from his written statement:

"Having sinned against society as well as God I feel it my duty to confess my guilt to society with deep humiliation and sincere repentance and ask forgiveness for all my offences against my fellow men."

"My present unfortunate position is the result of an unhappy marriage."

In explanation of his motive, Dr. King wrote: "Miss Vandervoort and myself were greatly enamored of each other. Actions speak louder than words, and I knew that she loved me, and that I could not help loving her in return. She was both lovely and loving. I looked upon her with all her personal charms, and attracting graces and virtues, her attainments and literary acquirements, her mild and affectionate disposition, her genial smiles and affable manners, her good character and winning ways, and while she perfectly reciprocated all my affections, it was as impossible for me not to love her as it would be to fly to the moon.

"Here then, I had found the object of my affections and the next thing was to get possession of that precious gem I had found, but there presented one obstacle in the way — my wife. It was only now that I allowed the thoughts to enter my mind of doing anything to shorten her life."

William further rationalized his actions by writing, "The law may compel man and wife to live together, but I defy it to compel them to love each other. Oh! how lamentable beyond description that so much misery and unhappiness should arise from unhappy marriages."

William refuted the experts' theories that his wife had died from the cumulative results of arsenic poisoning. He claimed he had given her chloroform. In describing his wife's last moments after she had fallen into a deep coma, he wrote: "Now I would have given worlds to have brought her to. I tried everything but could not succeed. O! what an awful feeling I then felt. How I repented, but, alas, it was too late. I just began to realize what had been done. Oh! the bitter pangs that I experienced cannot be imagined. The Devil had led me headlong into difficulty, but now came the remorse of conscience. Oh! how sharp, how pungent! I felt like death, and thought I would die."

Dr. King wasn't above passing out some free advice,

"The way to avoid trouble is not to get in. Better far, not to marry at all than to do so to your sorrow. To those who are married my parting advice is to pray to God for grace to guard you against all manner of temptation. Love your wives if you can possibly do so and use them kindly and affectionately if you can; but both men and women have their proper spheres in this life and sometimes they get united and there is no harmony in the family circle; if you cannot love your wives my advice to you is to separate, for you will either do one of two things; viz: be tempted to commit a crime perhaps that was the most foreign to your mind before, and that may force you first into jail, then in the criminal box to be put on trial for your life and have the sentence of death passed on you and thence face the halter and die a violent ignominious death amid a congregated multitude and go to a premature grave, or, you will be compelled to live a life of torture and drag out a miserable existence."

June 9, 1859 rolled around all too soon for Dr. King. He arose at 4 a.m. and ate a hearty breakfast. He then spent some time in prayer with Rev. Vanderburg. Several doctors who were close friends of the condemned man visited the jail to pay their respects. The solemn procession of jailers and spiritual advisors made its way to the scaffold. A crowd, estimated to be as high as 10,000, had trudged by foot and buggy to take in the spectacle. The public hanging took place without incident and the crowd dispersed.

Melinda Vandervoort took up with a new beau in Cleveland, but soon tired of him in favor of a gentleman from Montreal. Evidently, he left her high and dry in Montreal, after which she returned to Brighton, where she lived for many years, an object of scorn to many of the residents who knew her story. She drank heavily and is reported to have died in the late 1890s, penniless and alone, in an asylum in Toronto.

DR. THOMAS SMETHURST
1859

After a lengthy period of time, it is a rare crime that continues to hold the essential elements of mystery, intrigue and, above all, the burning question of the accused's innocence or guilt.

It is 134 years since Dr. Thomas Smethurst's star shone ever so brightly on the stage of murderous infamy. The good doctor was not a big man, nor was he particularly attractive. His one outstanding feature was his luxuriant crop of red hair. While still a student, Thomas met and married Mary Durham, who was a mature 51 and twenty years his senior. From the outset, there is no evidence that the doctor and his wife had anything but a conventional marriage.

Dr. Smethurst obtained his medical degree from the University of Erlangen and practised for years in both London and Ramsgate before selling his practice in 1853. For the next six years, he travelled extensively on the continent and in general, we are safe in assuming, led the good life.

In 1859, Thomas and Mary were living in quarters in a Bayswater rooming house. It was here that Thomas met Isabella Bankes, a fellow roomer. Let's consider Isabella's balance sheet for a moment. She was single, rather attractive in a delicate sort of way, was pleasant company, had a substantial income and was a relatively young 42. All of these assets compared favorably with Mrs. Smethurst, who had seen 74 summers come and go.

Ask any accountant; every balance sheet has some liabilities. Isabella had one flaw. She was subject to stomach trouble and often had to leave the dining room table to vomit. There is some evidence that this condition ran in the woman's family.

Isabella was charmed by the glib medic and there is little doubt that she fell in love. The basis of Thomas' attraction to Isabella was not as clear cut or well defined. We do know that the couple carried on to such an extent that the landlady of the rooming house, Mrs. Smith, asked Isabella to leave the premises.

Mrs. Smith must have mulled over in her mind the moral dilemma of a married man and a single woman hugging and kissing each other in front of other guests in her house against the loss of income if she tossed Miss Bankes out on her ear. The morals of the era won out. Isabella left. A short time later, Dr. Smethurst joined her. What Mrs. Smethurst thought of all this is unknown. It is a possibility that she was not aware of the other woman in her husband's life. Isn't it an axiom of the triangle business that the wife is always the last to know?

Dr. Thomas Smethurst and Isabella Bankes were married at Battersea Church and set up housekeeping in Richmond. It is inconceivable that Isabella wasn't aware that the man she was marrying was already married. Sly dogs in murderous plots have been known to pull off such deceptions, but on balance, Isabella simply had to know.

It wasn't long after the wedding that Isabella started to feel ill, which wasn't at all surprising. She had never been what you would call a healthy woman. Dr. Smethurst ministered to his new wife, but when she displayed a decided lack of improvement, he called in another doctor on the recommendation of his landlady, Mrs. Robinson.

Dr. Julius conferred with Smethurst and Isabella. He learned that she was suffering from excessive vomiting and diarrhea. He prescribed bismuth and common grey powder. When Isabella not only showed no improvement, but grew steadily worse, Dr. Julius suspected that somehow his patient was suffering from irritant poisoning. Dr. Julius called in his associate, Dr. Bird, to see Isabella. After Dr. Julius advised Dr. Bird of his suspicions, Dr. Bird agreed that the patient may have been poisoned.

It was seventeen days after Dr. Julius was first brought into the case that Dr. Smethurst called on a Richmond lawyer. On April 30, he showed up at the office of lawyer Senior with Isabella's will. It was handwritten by Smethurst. He suggested that Senior witness the signing the next day and do whatever lawyers do to make the will binding and legal. The following day, Senior called at the Smethursts', where he executed a proper will signed by Isabella Bankes, leaving her entire estate to Thomas Smethurst. She signed the will Isabella Bankes, not Isabella Smethurst, which leads one to believe that she knew very well she had taken part in a bigamous marriage.

While all this was going on, Isabella's health continued to deteriorate. The team of Julius and Bird called in yet another physician, Dr. Todd. He suggested that there was a real possibility that the patient was being poisoned and ordered that a stool be examined. This specimen was tested by Dr. Alfred Taylor, professor of chemistry at Guy's Hospital and a well known authority on such matters.

On May 2, 1859, based on this renowned doctor's findings, Dr. Smethurst was arrested and charged with administering poison. Dr. Smethurst told the court that his wife might die because of his absence. The presiding magistrate listened to his plea and released the prisoner on his own recognizance, but not before officials accompanied him to his home and confiscated all the bottles, vials and containers they could find. These were turned over to Dr. Taylor for examination. Next day, Isabella Bankes died. Dr. Taylor advised authorities that he had found arsenic in one of the bottles turned over to him for analysis. Dr. Smethurst was arrested and charged with murder.

In the years since Dr. Smethurst stood trial in London's Old Bailey, it is doubtful if any of the succeeding trials held there were more interesting or controversial than the Smethurst trial.

The prosecution contended that Isabella Bankes' death had been the culmination of an elaborate plot. As proof of this they produced a letter written by the accused man to his legal wife, telling her that it was his wish to be reunited with her and that it wouldn't be long before his wish would be fulfilled.

The fact that Dr. Smethurst stood to gain financially by Isabella's death weighed heavily against him. Isabella owned a property valued at £1800 which was left outright to Smethurst. However, the interest on £5000 she had been collecting ceased upon her death and reverted to other members of her family. Most sensational of all was the autopsy result. At the time of her death, Isabella was five to seven weeks pregnant.

An array of doctors took the witness stand for the prosecution, attesting to the state of Miss Bankes' internal organs. All agreed that the condition of these organs was compatible with irritant poisoning and nothing else.

It was left to Dr. Alfred Taylor, far and away the leading authority at the trial, to cause the greatest sensation and, some would say, embarrassment to the medical profession. Dr. Taylor stated that he had found no arsenic in any of Miss Bankes' internal organs. Under cross examination, he admitted that his previous statement given to a magistrate that he had found arsenic in one of the bottles seized on the day Smethurst was arrested was erroneous. Dr. Taylor said that a mistake had been made. He told the court that when he gave his original statement, he believed it to be true. Since then, he had discovered that while performing the tests for arsenic in that particular bottle he had used a copper gauze containing impurities which, in effect, had produced arsenic.

This was an explosive admission. Possession of poison is one of the salient elements in gaining convictions in poison cases. It was Dr. Taylor's original statement which had led to Dr. Smethurst being tried for murder. Now this vital piece of evidence had been revoked.

To be fair, as soon as he became aware of his grave error, Dr. Taylor had informed both the prosecution and the defence. In subsequent testimony, Dr. Taylor told the court that he had discovered minute quantities of antimony in one of the deceased woman's organs. One suspects that those in court wondered if the doctor hadn't made another mistake. Despite Dr. Taylor's error, other doctors swore that the condition of Isabella's organs could have been caused only by irritant poisoning.

The defence claimed that the Crown had not proven that Dr. Smethurst was in possession of either arsenic or antimony, nor had it proven that he had administered the deadly poison. They went on to point out that cutting off his rights to the interest on Isabella's £5000 was not the action of a man who killed for financial gain. As for the £1800 left to him, this sum would eventually have been his had Miss Bankes lived. The defence professed that, taking everything into consideration, Smethurst would have been better off financially had Miss Bankes not died. Then there was Miss Bankes' history of bilious attacks, general delicate health and pregnancy to consider.

To substantiate their claim, the defence paraded to the witness stand a distinguished group of doctors who swore that, in their opinion, after examining all the facts, Isabella had not been murdered, but had died of natural causes. Of the seventeen doctors who were called to the stand during the trial, ten claimed the victim was poisoned, while seven stated that she had died of natural causes.

The English jury deliberated only forty minutes before finding Dr. Smethurst guilty of murdering Isabella Bankes. The presiding judge expressed his agreement with the jury's verdict before passing the death sentence.

Once the verdict was made public, both the legal and medical communities challenged the justification for the death sentence. While all agreed that the doctor was a first class cad and might very well have killed his wife, they were adamant in their opinion that, based on the evidence, he should not have been convicted. Several expressed the opinion that even if conviction was warranted, the death sentence should not have been applied. Prestigious medical organizations wrote to officials stating their objections to the conviction. One example, representative of many, appeared in the Dublin Medical Press. Dripping with sarcasm, it reads:

"So much for the position to which the members of the medical profession, in their capacity as witnesses in criminal trials, have been degraded by Drs. Todd, Taylor, Julius, Bird, and Co. They have not left behind them one fixed opinion to guide the public press. The man who, par excellence, was looked upon as the pillar of medical jurisprudence; the man who it was believed could clear up the most obscure case, involving medico-legal considerations, ever brought into a court of justice; the man without whose assistance no criminal suspected of poisoning could be found guilty in England; the man whose opinion was quoted as the highest of all authorities at every trial where analysis is required, is the same who has now admitted the use of impure copper in an arsenic test where a life hung upon his evidence, the same who has brought an amount of disrepute upon his branch of the profession that years will not remove, the ultimate effects of which it is impossible to calculate, which none can regret with a deeper feeling of sorrow than ourselves, though, perhaps, in the end, a lesson may be taught which will not be lost upon the medical jurists, and which may tend to keep the fountain of justice clear and unpolluted. We must look now upon Professor Taylor as having ended his career, and hope he will immediately withdraw into the obscurity of private life, not forgetting to carry with him his favorite arsenical copper. He can never again be listened to in a court of justice, and should henceforth leave the witness-box to the occupation of others."

Scores of such documents were forwarded to the Home Secretary, who in turn sent all the documents, several of them learned treatises on the subject of poisons and the condition of Miss Bankes' internal organs, to Sir Benjamin Collins Brodie, the most prominent medical authority in England. Dr. Brodie studied all the material and came to the conclusion that although the medical evidence threw suspicion on Dr. Smethurst, there was no positive proof of his guilt. As a result of this report, it was suggested to Queen Victoria that she take the rare step of granting Dr. Smethurst a free pardon. The Queen took the advice and the doctor was freed.

Dr. Smethurst wasn't totally out of the woods. In November 1859, he was charged with bigamy, found guilty and sentenced to one year in prison at hard labor. The man of medicine served his time. Two years after his release, he took legal action to collect on Isabella Bankes' will. The court ruled the document valid. Dr. Thomas Smethurst collected the proceeds of Isabella's will.

DR. EDMUND POMMERAIS
1863

I have always been a firm believer that one day a year should be set aside for mothers-in-law. Despite common belief, mothers-in-law, as a class, can be a fine group of ladies. Unfortunately, as individuals, they can be extremely annoying. What's even more exasperating, they are usually correct in their opinions.

Let's go back a few years across the big pond to meet Madame Dubizy and her future son-in-law, Edmund Pommerais, of Paris, France.

We'll start with Edmund, just for fun.

Ed was a tall, handsome lad of 24 when he arrived on the Parisian scene in 1860. Like many freshly turned out doctors, our boy thought it would be commendable to heal those on the bottom rung of the economic ladder. Before you could say syringe, Dr. Pommerais had a huge practice of non-paying, poor, sick patients.

This would have been just fine if the doctor hadn't had such expensive tastes. Ed was somewhat of a dandy when it came to clothing. He also maintained a lavishly furnished apartment and, in general, threw money around like it was going out of style. As his debts rose, so did his longing for female companionship. Just when the doctor felt those old biological urges, who should come strolling into his clinic but Madame Seraphine de Pauw. The poorly dressed but attractive lady had a husband in dire need of Dr. Pommerais' skill. Ed was more than willing to take on yet one more impoverished patient. Sadly, I must relate that despite the doctor's loving care, Mr. de Pauw was carried away to his great reward after several months.

Now, Madame de Pauw was ten years older than the doctor. Besides, she was encumbered with three small children, but as we all know, love or sex or whatever is blind. Madame de Pauw became Ed's mistress. Although deeply in debt, Ed managed to provide for her and the children.

Nothing wrong with all that, you might say, but darn it all, the bills kept mounting up. Ed was desperately in debt when, quite by chance, he met Madame Dubizy, who came complete with charming daughter. Ed did a double take. Dubizy was an old battle-axe, but the daughter was built like one of those sexy manikins on display at Galleries Lafayette.

When Ed found out that the Dubizy clan was loaded with francs, he decided to woo and wed Dubizy the younger. Despite the madame's open dislike for our Ed, he managed to court and finally marry her young daughter.

That's when Madame Dubizy showed her true colors. She fixed up her daughter's wealth so that Ed could not get his hands on any of it. That is, as long as Madame Dubizy lived. Ed made a mental note that it might not be that long.

Ed was a busy boy. Of necessity, he had to break the news of his marriage to Seraphine de Pauw and let her know that their private horizontal arrangements would have to undergo something of an adjustment. Seraphine sobbed, but Ed assured her he would send her enough cash to keep the wolf from the door. Let's give Ed his due — he sent a few francs for a couple of months. Then he quit. Out of sight, out of mind.

Ed was putting out fires as fast as they broke out, but there was one blaze he couldn't quell. Those enormous debts kept piling up. Since he insisted that his wife have the best clothing and jewelry, his marriage, rather than alleviating his precarious position, only served to add to it.

That's when he decided to kill his mother-in-law. It wasn't that difficult. One evening Ed and the wife had dear Mama over for dinner. Ed liberally laced her favorite wine with poison. An hour after quaffing back half a litre, Mama felt ill. Not to worry. After all, her son-in-law was a doctor. Ed stayed with his stricken mother-in-law until dawn. Then he broke the sad news to his wife. Mama had departed this mortal coil.

Solicitous Ed comforted his wife, made all the funeral arrangements and signed the death certificate. He then got his grubby little paws on his mother-in-law's estate. The total amount conveniently wiped out Ed's enormous debts. Mama's death couldn't have been more timely.

Ed continued on his merry way. He gambled heavily on the stock market and lived lavishly. It was only a matter of months before he was once again over his head in debt. He attempted to borrow money through legitimate channels, but no bank would take a chance on him. Desperately, he tried money lenders, but they too wouldn't have any part of a man so deeply in the red.

At this juncture in Ed's life, who should write him a letter but Seraphine de Pauw. Seraphine could tear your heart out. She and her children lived in a hovel and were literally starving to death. She apologized for bothering Ed, but if there was anything he could do, it sure would be appreciated. Ed dropped in on his old flame. The situation was just as Seraphine had outlined in her letter. Ed produced 20 francs for food and became an instant hero to Seraphine and the children.

In the following days, Ed once more entered his old girlfriend's life. The flame, which had diminished over the years, once more burned brightly. Seraphine figured her lover was loaded. Quite the opposite was true. Ed was dead broke and was delicately perched on the edge of bankruptcy and ruin. He did, however, have a diabolical plan.

He persuaded Seraphine, now completely under his influence, to take out a large insurance policy on her life. The face value was the equivalent of $150,000, a magnificent sum in the mid-nineteenth century. Ed would pay the first year's premium. Seraphine would then fake illness and call in her doctor, namely Edmund Pommerais. Ed would inform the insurance boys that their policy holder would be occupying a plot at the local cemetery within 12 months. Cunning Ed told Seraphine that the insurance company would offer her a cash settlement in order to avoid paying off the higher amount on her death. Ed explained that once they got their hands on the settlement money, they would be able to continue their relationship in style.

Seraphine de Pauw looked at the handsome young doctor who had re-entered her life like Prince Charming. She would do anything he asked. When Ed explained that he might have to give her some nasty medicine, which would make her feel slightly ill for a few days, she understood. After all, another doctor might be called in and it would be necessary to deceive him. Naturally, Ed was the beneficiary on the policy. To be on the safe side, he had Seraphine sign a will leaving everything to him. The poor woman had no idea what she was signing.

Ed's diabolical plot was put into motion. He scraped up the money to pay the first year's premium. Seraphine purchased the life insurance policy. After waiting a few months, she pretended to faint in front of neighbors in her tenement building. The rumor spread that she was in failing health. Finally, after one particular fainting spell, a neighbor called the doctor. Quick as a bunny, Ed was on the scene. He gave his patient some medicine, which contained small quantities of poison.

In the following days, neighbors visited. No question about it, Seraphine was seriously ill. Each day, Dr. Pommerais made a house call. Nothing seemed to help.

While Seraphine suffered, she firmly believed that her discomfort would soon be over and yield her a fortune. During a visit from her sister, Madame Ritter, Seraphine confided that her sickness was a sham. She told her sister the entire scheme. The story was so convincing, Madame Ritter believed it and told no one.

On November 17, 1863, Seraphine de Pauw died in agony. A neighbor called Dr. Pommerais. The doctor was at his lover's side during her final moments.

Ed wasn't a patient man. He was just itching to get his hands on that insurance money. He waited a week. On the day after Seraphine's funeral, he applied for the pay-off. The insurance company acknowledged the claim and were about to issue a cheque, when who should show up but Madame Ritter with her unusual story.

Well, folks, the fat was in the fire. Seraphine de Pauw's body was exhumed and found to contain large quantities of digitaline. Ed was arrested and taken into custody. Madame Dubizy's body was also exhumed, but the exact cause of death could not be found. It didn't matter much.

Ed stood accused of murder. At his trial, Madame Ritter's story was enough to convince the jury that Ed had indeed murdered Seraphine de Pauw.

Dr. Edmund Pommerais was executed for his crime. He vehemently protested his innocence to the end. No one believed him.

DR. EDWARD PRITCHARD
1865

Dr. Edward Pritchard married Miss Mary Jane Taylor in 1850 and, after accepting various medical posts, settled down to his own private practice in Glasgow, Scotland.

Now Dr. Pritchard was a tall, sensitive, attractive man, with a full flowing beard. He was extremely popular with his patients, but when it came to female patients, there were gossips who spread the word. It seems the good doctor performed extensive examinations on attractive ladies, when perhaps a more cursory examination would have sufficed. The doctor loved to spend money and loved to have a good time. He was a real charmer. However, this charm did not carry over to his professional colleagues. They frowned on the low standard of medicine he practised, and his private life.

All went well at home until May of 1863, when unaccountably a fire broke out in the servants' quarters of the Pritchard home. Mrs. Pritchard and another servant were out of town at the time. When firemen put out the blaze, the body of a young servant girl was found burned to death in her bed. She had made no attempt to leave the bed. It was one of those minor mysteries that occurs in every large city. While a few suspicious glances were tossed the doctor's way, nothing was ever done about it.

The experience was so distasteful the family moved to Clarence Place, and then things started to happen. The new home was four storeys high. The doctor and his wife lived in apparent harmony with four of their five children. The oldest lived with her grandparents in Edinburgh. The Pritchards had two servants, the cook, Catherine Lattimer, and Mary M'leod, a maid who was hired to replace the poor unfortunate servant who was burned in her bed.

Mary herself got burned in bed, after a fashion. You see, she and the doctor had arrived at an understanding that was not exactly the normal master-servant relationship. Mary became pregnant. Edward hastily performed an operation on Mary which had the desired effect of producing a miscarriage. After a brief recovery period, Mary and Dr. Pritchard continued their illicit relationship.

In October 1864, Mrs. Pritchard, who was always a robust healthy woman, started to suffer from headaches and stomach cramps. It got so bad, her husband confined her to bed. Her mother, Mrs. Taylor, wrote from Edinburgh that her daughter should visit with her to regain her health. At first the doctor wouldn't hear of being parted from his wife. Finally he yielded under pressure, and Mrs. Pritchard went to her mother's home. Here her health improved dramatically and rapidly.

On December 22, Mrs. Pritchard came home to be with her family for Christmas. Almost immediately, she became ill again. She was vomiting after every meal. She became so violently ill that late in January, Dr. Pritchard wrote his wife's cousin, one Dr. Cowan, in Edinburgh, to come and visit Mrs. Pritchard. On February 7, Dr. Cowan arrived and applied a mustard poultice to his cousin. Upon his return to Edinburgh he urged Mrs. Taylor to go to Glasgow to attend her daughter. In the meantime, Mrs. Pritchard had her worst attack to date. Despite her husband, who stood at her bedside, she implored the cook to fetch Dr. Gairdner, who lived close by. When he arrived he was told by Dr. Pritchard that Dr. Cowan had given his wife stimulants. Dr. Gairdner suggested this be stopped immediately. He prescribed a simple diet, and next day he was advised that Mrs. Pritchard was much better. Despite this reassurance, Dr. Gairdner became apprehensive about the entire matter. He remembered that Mrs. Pritchard's brother was also a doctor. They had attended college together. He wrote Dr. Taylor, who in turn wrote to his brother-in-law and suggested that it might be best if his sister visited him. Dr. Pritchard wouldn't hear of being parted from his dear wife.

In the meantime Mrs. Taylor came to Glasgow to be with her daughter. She found her continuously vomiting and suffering from severe cramps. Within a week Mrs. Taylor started to feel ill. On the night of February 16, she became so violently sick she was placed in bed with her daughter. Dr. Pritchard called another neighbor who was also a man of medicine, Dr. James Patterson.

If you are keeping score, this is the fourth doctor called in to treat one or the other of the two very sick ladies. Not counting Dr. Pritchard's ministrations, the total medical treatment up to this time was one mustard poultice, applied to Mrs. Pritchard. However, one must keep in mind that all the doctors were dealing with another doctor, who was the husband and son-in-law of the patients.

When Dr. Patterson entered the house, he was greeted by Dr. Pritchard and given the usual misleading symptoms. Upon examining Mrs. Taylor, Dr. Patterson gave the opinion that she was under the influence of dope, probably opium, and was dying of opiate poisoning. He said there was nothing he could do. At 11:30 p.m. he left the house. At 1 a.m. he got a call to return but refused, saying that death was inevitable. Mrs. Taylor passed away a few minutes after 1 a.m. Dr. Pritchard signed the death certificate "paralysis 12 hours. Apoplexy one hour."

Dr. Pritchard continued to supervise everything consumed by his wife who deteriorated rapidly. Finally on Friday, March 17, after four months of excruciating pain, attended by her husband and Dr. Patterson, Mrs. Pritchard passed away. During her final hours Patterson asked Pritchard to make up a simple sleeping draught, but Pritchard replied that he kept no drugs in the house.

Dr. Pritchard was again called upon to sign a death certificate. This time he wrote "gastric fever, two months."

On Monday, March 20, Mr. William Hart, who held a post roughly equivalent to that of our coroner, received an anonymous letter. In substance it told of the two deaths and suggested foul play may have been involved. When the doctor arrived back in Glasgow from his wife's funeral in Edinburgh, he was detained by the police. Routine investigation revealed his relationship with Mary M'Leod. To make matters worse it was revealed that poor Mrs. Pritchard had stumbled on her husband and Mary in sundry compromising positions. She had long before decided to sidestep a scandal, and put up with her promiscuous husband and maid. The bodies of Mrs. Pritchard and her mother were exhumed, and found to be full of poison.

Edward Pritchard was arrested and stood trial for murder on Monday, July 3, 1865. While his trial caused a sensation, it provided no duelling match between prosecution and defence attorneys. There was really no defence. For a man who professed to have no drugs in his home, his two suppliers provided a list of drugs purchased by the physician during his victims' illness. They included enough poison to do away with half of dear old Glasgow.

Through it all the doctor remained a charming, polite scoundrel. He was found guilty and sentenced to hang. Before he was led to the scaffold in the presence of an Episcopalian minister, he confessed to both murders "in the way brought out in the evidence." Monster that he was, he kept his charming charade to the very end. Head erect, with a bold, almost marching step, he was hanged before a huge crowd on July 28, 1865.

Handsome Edward had the distinction to be the last person to be publicly executed in Glasgow.

DR. GEORGE LAMSON
1882

To perform murder in Victorian England and have the case still considered to be a classic is no mean feat. In those days young people often died due to maladies caused by unsanitary conditions, contaminated water, and tainted food. Those who didn't die of natural causes were often eased into oblivion with the help of some poison or other which was not readily detected. An innovative approach was required to stand out in such a crowd.

Dr. George Lamson was such a trail blazer. At the age of 20 he was studying medicine in Paris. In 1878, by the time he was 28, he was practising medicine in London, England, and had taken a wife.

Pretty Kate John was everything a Victorian wife should have been—pleasant, gracious, devoted, and loyal to her handsome, educated husband. Kate's younger brother, Hubert, died of natural causes a year after the couple's marriage. This tragedy did have a silver lining. Hubert left the Lamsons an amount of money which enabled the good doctor to purchase a medical practice in Bournemouth.

Kate had another brother, Percy. Sixteen-year-old Percy had curvature of the spine, which left him paralyzed from the waist down. Confined to a wheelchair, he was placed in a private school, Blenheim House in Wimbledon, where he seemed to fit in well with the other boys.

All went well for some time. Being a doctor, and husband to a woman who deeply cared for her afflicted brother, it was only natural that Dr. Lamson displayed a certain concern for Percy. On December 3, 1881, he visited Blenheim House.

The principal of the school, William Bedbrook, fetched Percy when the doctor arrived. Dr. Lamson had brought some treats. From a black bag he produced some hard fruit candy and a fruitcake. The doctor cut the cake with a penknife, offering a slice to Percy and the principal, as well as taking a slice himself. All three almost finished the cake at the one sitting.

During the course of idle conversation, Dr. Lamson mentioned that he had recently returned from America and had brought back something new—gelatin capsules. The gelatin dissolved after the capsule was swallowed, effectively doing away with the disagreeable taste of some medicines. Both the principal and Percy tried one. The principal's was empty, but Percy's was filled with sugar from a sugar bowl sitting on a table nearby. He swallowed it without tasting the sugar at all.

The doctor terminated his visit and left the school, informing the principal that he had to catch a train later that night for Florence.

That evening Percy complained of heartburn and went to bed. Later he began to vomit and convulse violently. Two doctors were summoned, but they could do nothing for the boy. At 11:20 that same evening Percy died.

On December 6, a post mortem was held, and it was the opinion of the doctors that Percy had been poisoned. Dr. Lamson was located in Paris. Once informed of the death in the family he immediately returned to London. By that time the story of his visit to the school was known to the authorities. He was arrested and charged with murder.

On March 8, 1882, Lamson's murder trial began in London's Old Bailey. The prosecution quickly established that Percy had been done in by aconite, one of the most lethal poisons known to man. Dr. Lamson had purchased aconite shortly before his visit to the school. He also was deeply in debt and stood to gain financially from Percy's death.

In all murder cases involving poison, the prosecution must establish that the victim was in fact poisoned, and that the accused administered the poison. It was this second point that proved to be a sticky wicket. Bedbrook, the principal, was present at all times during Lamson's visit. The hard candies weren't touched. All three ate the cake. The sugar, which went into the capsule consumed by Percy, came from the school's own sugar bowl.

Despite this little problem, and the doctor's insistence throughout that he was innocent, he was found guilty and sentenced to hang. The sentence was carried out on April 28, 1882. The day before he was hanged Dr. Lamson confessed in writing to the murder of his brother-in-law. He never did state how he had administered the poison, and the solution to the case has baffled criminologists down through the years.

Here is the diabolical method most accepted by those who have closely studied the case. The speculation is that the doctor injected aconite into a raisin, which he then placed back into the cake. He marked the part of the cake containing the fatal raisin, making sure he gave the piece to his victim.

DR. PHILIP CROSS
1887

Dr. Philip Cross surveyed his domain from his fine old home in Dripson, Ireland. The doctor had recently retired from the British Army after serving for many years in India. Now in the winter of 1886 the old man could look forward to many peaceful, if not somewhat boring, years with his wife, Laura, his children, at his retirement estate known as Shandy Hill.

It was not a future that promised much excitement, but many men work a lifetime for just such twilight years of contentment. The doctor was a gruff, introverted man who apparently tolerated the matronly Mrs. Cross as long as she conveniently stayed out of his way. Then again, the British Army does develop character.

When twenty-one-year-old Effie Skinner joined the staff of Shandy Hill as governess to the Cross children the doctor paid little attention. It is hard to believe the doctor ignored the new governess, for Effie was a peach. Her complexion was unblemished, and when she smiled, two pink dimples appeared on each cheek.

It is unclear exactly when the kindly doctor did take notice of this breath of spring. A smile, a touch, a hidden kiss, who knows? At first the embarrassed Effie rejected the doctor's advances. But old Dr. Phil slowly won Effie to his side both literally and figuratively. Stolen kisses in the hall of Shandy Hill led to more basic acts behind closed doors. Dr. Cross and Effie became lovers.

As was inevitable, Mrs. Cross found out about her husband's dalliance with the hired help. Laura could have become indignant, but instead, she decided to let bygones be bygones. After all, Phil had never before acted in this unfaithful manner. Mrs. Cross did the practical thing. She gave Effie her notice. This may not appear to be a major calamity today, but an unemployed governess without references before the turn of the century could end up begging on the street.

To the rescue came Dr. Cross. Effie was understandably grateful for any help. The doctor's proposition was simple enough. He would provide the necessary cash for a flat in Dublin and would visit his paramour at every opportunity. Effie became Dr. Cross' mistress.

This new and convenient arrangement went along famously for several months. There was just one thing. The spry old doctor was in love with Effie and wanted to be with her all the time. Meanwhile, back home at Shandy Hill, Mrs. Cross began to suffer from the most annoying stomach cramps. Sometimes her distress was so severe as to bring on attacks of vomiting. Phil ministered to his wife for several weeks before bringing in Dr. Godfrey, a cousin and friend of the family, for another opinion. Phil explained to his colleague that Laura was suffering from a slight attack of typhoid fever. Dr. Godfrey examined Mrs. Cross and quickly concurred with the older and more experienced doctor. After all, who would detect typhoid fever if not a former military doctor who had spent years in India?

On May 24, 1887, when the local clergyman Rev. Mr. Hayes called to pay his respects to the ill Mrs. Cross, he was told by the kindly doctor that she had just dropped off to sleep. A most distressing week passed for Mrs. Cross. She suffered greatly from nausea and vomiting. On June 2, the maid, Mary Buckley, was awakened by the frantic doctor. Mrs. Cross had mercifully passed away.

Dr. Cross signed the death certificate without delay. Mrs. Cross was laid to rest two days later. The brief ceremony, conducted at graveside at the ungodly hour of

6 a.m., was thought by some good citizens of Dripson to be decidedly odd. It mattered not what the Dripsonites thought, for Dr. Cross was off to his true love.

Like a man possessed, he gathered up Effie in Dublin and sped to London, where the older gentleman and the 21-year-old governess became man and wife. Dr. Phil and Effie tiptoed through the English countryside on their honeymoon. Back in Ireland news reached Dripson that the doctor had married the former governess, and only two weeks after Mrs. Cross had given up the ghost. A relative wrote Dr. Cross informing him that his friends and neighbors had not taken kindly to his actions. The doctor felt that he had better return to Shandy Hill for appearances' sake.

Once ensconced in his old home, the doctor kept a low profile. But nasty rumors failed to abate. There were those who remembered that Dr. Cross had tended to his wife in her final illness. Then there was the hasty funeral. Bad news travels fast. It wasn't long before Inspector Tyacke of the Royal Irish Constabulary heard the rumors.

The inspector spoke to the coroner, who felt there was enough monkey business taking place to order an inquest. In conjunction with the inquest Mrs. Cross' body was exhumed. An autopsy indicated that she had never had so much as a touch of typhoid fever. What she did have was a massive quantity of arsenic, accounting for the nausea and vomiting she suffered before death.

Dr. Phil was arrested and charged with the murder of his first wife. He didn't have a chance. The prosecution produced one of those chemists who have a habit of taking the witness stand and pointing at the accused. The motive — Effie — was there for all to see.

On January 10, 1888, Dr. Cross, whose hair, incidentally, had turned chalk white during his confinement, was hanged for the murder of his wife.

DR. NEILL CREAM
1890

The 1920s have often been referred to as the golden age of sport. Babe Ruth was clouting home runs, while Jack Dempsey was clouting anyone who stood in his way.

In the murder business the period between 1880 and 1895 should be called the Golden Age of Mayhem. It gave rise to so many unusual murders. A chap known as Jack the Ripper was roaming the streets of London cutting up ladies of the night. On this side of the big pond, a God-fearing, church-going New England lady named Lizzie Borden was accused of chopping up her mummie and daddy with a hatchet.

With the murder stage being so crowded with nefarious players, it is no wonder that Dr. Neill Cream never gained the notoriety he so richly deserved.

Neill was born in Glasgow, Scotland in 1850. His family migrated to Canada when he was five. Nothing is known of his formative years other than that he applied himself diligently to his schoolwork and did exceedingly well throughout high school. He continued on to McGill University in Montreal, where he received his medical degree. He later took post graduate work in London and Edinburgh before returning to Canada.

For the next five years Neill Cream led an eventful, if somewhat jaded existence. He set up practice in various Canadian towns and cities, but was always forced to stay on the move. You see, Dr. Cream's medical standards were decidedly below the norm, particularly when he was examining female patients. In fact, it wasn't an uncommon sight to see a lady running out of Dr. Cream's office in a state of undress. Finally, he found the temperature so unbearably hot that he left Canada for Chicago, in order to have more freedom to practise his particular brand of medicine.

In 1881, Dr. Cream went too far. He gave a huge quantity of strychnine to a patient named Stott. It is believed that the motive was two fold. Stott had a pretty wife whom the doctor was examining all the time, although her neighbors later stated that this was very strange since she was never sick a day in her life. It is believed to this day that Mrs. Stott was involved with Cream in her husband's sudden demise. At the time of Stott's death, Cream was trying to place a large insurance policy on the unfortunate man's life, with himself as the beneficiary.

Stott's death at first was attributed to natural causes. Then Dr. Cream did an extraordinary thing, which he continued to do throughout his criminal career. He started writing letters. He wrote to both the coroner and the district attorney suggesting that Stott's body be exhumed. Finally, at the anonymous urging of Cream the body was disinterred. Upon examination, it was found to be chock full of strychnine.

Dr. Cream and Mrs. Stott took off, but were soon apprehended and indicted for murder. Mrs. Stott, cutie that she was, testified for the state. Charges against her were dropped. Dr. Cream was found guilty of second degree murder and was sentenced to life imprisonment. In 1881, the prison gates of Joliet closed behind the strange doctor, but his career was far from over. In 1891, after Cream had spent just under 10 years in prison, Gov. Fifer of Illinois commuted his sentence, and Neill Cream walked out of prison, a free man. The governor had made a horrendous error.

While he had been spending time in prison, Cream's father died, leaving him an inheritance of $16,000, a veritable fortune before the turn of the century. Dr. Cream picked up the cash and headed for England, arriving in

London on October 1, 1891. Whether it was the London fog or whatever, Dr. Cream didn't waste any time pursuing his secondary occupation, that of poisoner.

A 19-year-old prostitute, Ellen Donworth, let herself be picked up by Cream. During the course of the evening her tall, austere looking friend, sporting a top hat, offered her a drink out of his flask. She took two long drags of the bottle and almost immediately began to suffer from convulsions. Her friend was nowhere to be found, but neighbors called a doctor, who rushed the girl to the hospital. She died en route. An autopsy revealed that Ellen had died of strychnine poisoning.

The police had no clues to the poisoner's identity, but never fear. Our Dr. Cream made sure that he received some of the recognition he craved. He wrote the coroner offering to reveal the killer's identity in return for £200,000. The letter was signed A. O'Brien. The coroner tried to set up a rendezvous, but O'Brien-Cream never showed up.

One week after the Donworth murder, another prostitute, Matilda Clover, was found in her room writhing in agony. Her client for the evening, a man who called himself Fred, had given her some pills. Before she died, she described Fred to a friend who lived in the same house. Fred was a tall, well-built man, who dressed in a cape and tall silk hat. For some reason, Matilda's death was thought to have been caused by alcoholism, but Cream would have none of it. He dashed off a note to a distinguished doctor, accusing him of poisoning Matilda with strychnine. The doctor took the letter to the police. Other distinguished people received letters accusing them of poisoning Matilda. Because of the veritable shower of letters, Matilda's body was exhumed. The cause of her death was attributed to strychnine. Scotland Yard now realized that a systematic killer was on the loose in London.

The winter months drifted by without any further

murders at the hands of the mysterious poisoner, with an abnormal urge for revealing his crimes in letters. Later, when every move Cream made was reviewed, the reason he stopped poisoning prostitutes during the winter months became clear. He had taken a trip to Canada, where strangely enough, he had printed 500 circulars, a copy of which follows:

ELLEN DONWORTH'S DEATH

To the Guests of the Metropole Hotel. Ladies and Gentlemen:

I hereby notify you that the person who poisoned Ellen Donworth on the 13th last October is today in the employ of the Metropole Hotel and that your lives are in danger as long as you remain in this Hotel. London April 1892.

Yours respectfully,

W.H. Murray

Dr. Cream never used the printed circulars, and no one knows to this day why he had them printed. They do serve to reveal Cream's perverted obsession with publicity of any kind.

With the coming of spring, and with Cream back in England, things started to percolate once again.

Emma Shrivell, an 18-year-old prostitute and her friend, Alice March, lived in a furnished flat near Waterloo Road. In the middle of the night their screams woke the landlady. Both girls were in great pain and were convulsing violently. During brief periods when their agony subsided, they told of having a distinguished gentleman as a supper guest earlier that evening. The gentleman wore a tall top hat, called himself Fred, and claimed he was a doctor. The girls let him talk them into taking some pills. Alice March died before reaching the hospital, while Emma Shrivell lingered for five hours before she too died.

Quite by chance a bobby walking his beat had seen the two girls let their guest out into the night. He was able to provide a full description. The publicity surrounding these two deaths brought forth other ladies who had managed to escape the clutches of the mysterious Fred.

Lou Harvey told of pretending to take the pills, but unknown to Fred she had thrown them away. Violet Beverley refused a drink offered to her by the obliging Fred. Both of these ladies gave detailed descriptions of their weird acquaintance to the police.

Then Dr. Cream, still craving notoriety, did the ultimate. He complained to Scotland Yard. Using the name Dr. Neill, he told them that the police were following him and harassing him with accusations that he was the killer of March and Shrivell. Neill told the Yard that he had nothing whatever to do with the crimes, claiming that a Dr. Harper was the real culprit.

It is difficult to understand exactly why Dr. Cream would furnish the police with information which would lead them to his doorstep. It wasn't long before the authorities discovered that Dr. Neill was really Dr. Cream. Several of the surviving ladies identified him as the elusive Fred. So did the bobby who had seen him leave March and Shrivell's flat the night they died.

Dr. Cream was 42 years old when he was adjudged to be legally sane and placed on trial for murder. On November 15, 1892 he was hanged for his crimes.

With death only seconds away Cream's sense of the dramatic was not to be denied. As the trap door sprung open he yelled, "I am Jack the R—." Reporters ran to their files, only to find out that Dr. Cream had been securely locked up in Joliet when Jack was operating in London.

Dr. Cream suffered his greatest indignity when more than 80 years after his execution, Madame Tussaud's wax museum in London announced they were removing his wax image from their Chamber of Horrors. It seems there was a decided lack of interest, and anyway he wasn't scary enough.

DR. ROBERT BUCHANAN
1891

Doctors should really stay out of the murder business and stick to healing. Don't get me wrong, as a class of killer, men of medicine can be extremely adept at sending the unsuspecting to the great hereafter, but for some reason, at the conclusion of the dastardly deed, they are prone to act in a downright stupid manner.

Dr. Robert Buchanan left Halifax, N.S. to set up his office in New York City. He and wife Helen settled at 267 West 11th St., where he gradually built up a rather lucrative practice.

Bob was not the robust swashbuckling type. He was a short man with a rather sad countenance set off by a scraggly moustache. He did have two outstanding traits. He loved the ladies and had a thirst that could only be quenched in the many saloons which dotted his neighborhood.

After living in New York for four years, Doc Bob was a regular patron at a saloon owned by Richard Macomber. He got to know Macomber and another regular, William Doria, extremely well. The three men downed many a slug of rotgut during the cold New York nights. Boys will be boys.

One night in 1890 the three friends ventured to Newark to visit a house of ill fame owned and operated by the partnership of madam Anna Sutherland and elderly janitor James Smith.

Can we take a moment here to describe Anna Sutherland? Just as the doctor's wife Helen was an attractive woman, Anna was not. She was fat, I mean really big.

She wore excessive makeup and dyed her hair a hideous shade of red. Unfortunately, she had a distinctive and prominent wart on her nose. Doc Bob was not yet 30; Anna was twice the good doctor's age.

When Doc Bob's two buddies tired of their periodic sojourns to Newark, the doctor continued to visit Anna. Soon he was taking care of her minor medical ills. Quite unexpectedly, Doc Bob informed his friends that he was divorcing Helen. He swore he was through with marriage. The divorce was granted on November 12, 1891. Exactly 14 days later, Anna Sutherland made out a will, leaving everything she owned to her future husband or, if she died single, to her dear friend, Dr. Bob Buchanan. Three days after she made out her will, Anna married Bob. Helen moved back to Halifax. Bob relocated his practice in Anna's brothel on Halsey St. in Newark.

Medicine and prostitution do not as a rule mix well. Male patients would often be accosted by Anna at the doctor's front door. She would inquire as to their preferences in a sex partner. This did nothing to enhance Doc Bob's medical practice. To make matters worse, James Smith, Anna's partner in the prostitution business, was extremely jealous of the doctor, whom he considered an interloper. After all, James had proposed more than once to Anna and had been turned down every time.

Folks, the marriage didn't work, but Doc Bob hung on until well into 1892. There is little doubt that the doctor put his plan into action in March of that year when he purchased a single ticket to Edinburgh to further his medical studies. The ticket was for travel on April 25. When Anna heard that she wasn't included in the trip, she threatened to cut him out of her will. On April 21, Doc Bob told his buddies down at the saloon that dear Anna had become too ill to travel and that he had cancelled the trip.

On April 22, Dr. B.C. McIntyre was called in to

minister to Anna. The doctor found Mrs. Buchanan raving and near hysteria. She complained that her throat was contracting. When his patient lapsed into a coma, Dr. McIntyre called in Dr. H.P. Watson for a second opinion. Next day, after an illness of only 26 hours, Anna died with both doctors in attendance. Death was attributed to a cerebral hemmorhage.

Dr. Bob displayed no sorrow at the loss of his wife. In fact, he was elated. Anna had left him a cool $50,000, an absolute fortune in those days. Bob took off for Halifax, but before he left he hired a private detective to guard his late wife's grave. That was a stupid thing to do.

Lurking in the reeds, observing everything through his beady eyes, was Anna's old partner, James Smith. That sterling gentleman smelled a rat and hightailed it to the coroner's office with his suspicions. The coroner listened, but upon learning that two reputable doctors had been at Anna's bedside throughout her illness, dismissed Smith as a troublemaker.

A reporter for the old New York World overheard the conversation and decided to look into Anna's untimely death. He dropped into Doc Bob's favorite watering hole and learned of the doctor's aborted trip to Scotland. He checked with the steamship company and learned that Bob had cancelled his passage and had obtained a refund on April 11, over a week before his wife had taken ill.

The reporter, now hot to trot, also learned that Doc Bob and his cronies had often discussed a current New York murder case which involved morphine. Doc Bob had expressed the opinion that he could administer a lethal dose of morphine which would never be detected. When the reporter learned that the doctor had remarried his first wife Helen in Halifax, he knew he was tracking down a diabolical killer.

The New York World put its case to the coroner who agreed to exhume Mrs. Buchanan's body. An autopsy revealed the presence of a residue of morphine, indicating that Anna had been given enough morphine to kill her. When the dead woman's eyes were checked for telltale contractions of the pupils (even after death an obvious symptom of morphine poisoning), doctors were shocked to note that there was no contraction.

The district attorney's office was convinced that Doc Bob had found a method of concealing this symptom. Someone in the DA's office remembered that, as a little boy, he had been given drops of belladonna to enlarge his pupils for an eye examination. Anna's eyeballs were tested for belladonna. Sure enough, they tested positive. When a nurse who had attended Anna before the two physicians arrived at the house recalled that Doc Bob had given his wife eye drops for no apparent reason, the doctor was arrested and taken into custody.

On March 20, 1893, Doc Bob stood trial for the murder of his wife. The evidence against him was entirely circumstantial. A strange demonstration took place in the courtroom. A cat was poisoned with morphine. Belladonna was dropped into the cat's eyes, which served to disguise the contraction of its pupils.

On April 26, the New York jury deliberated for 28 hours before returning a verdict of guilty of murder in the first degree. Dr. Robert Buchanan lingered on Sing Sing's Death Row for two years. On July 2, 1895, he was executed in the electric chair.

DR. HENRY MEYER
1894

Years ago groups of ambitious men sat around grog shops in London, England, betting on whether or not the latest explorer to the new world would make it back to England. From these humble beginnings sprang what we know today as the insurance business. Almost as quickly as the insurance industry developed, another group of cunning individuals developed schemes to defraud the insurance companies.

None was more cunning that Dr. Henry C. Meyer of Chicago. The good doctor had been in and out of trouble all of his adult life, having had the misfortune of having his first two wives die under mysterious circumstances. Was the man of medicine discouraged? Not on your life. He appeared before the altar for the third time in 1888 with a blue-eyed, rosy-cheeked young thing of 20, who sported long braids down to her waist. The doctor was 38.

Dr. Meyer had an unprofitable back-street practice and was struggling to make ends meet, when a patient, Ludwig Brandt, strolled into his office. Ludwig was to change Dr. Meyer's life forever.

Ludwig was in the insurance business. His conversation about claims and big payoffs simply fascinated Dr. Meyer. It seemed that a man with an overabundance of grey matter between his ears would have no trouble at all parting those wealthy insurance companies from some of their cash. A few months after their initial meeting the two men decided to defraud Ludwig's own company.

Ludwig had no trouble obtaining insurance on a nonexistent person. Dr. Meyer then produced a cadaver. Mrs. Meyer, posing as the cadaver's sister, would collect the insurance money. The scheme lacked sophistication, was amateurish, and fell apart when the examining physician made the startling discovery that the cadaver had been dead for some days rather than a few minutes.

To every cloud there is a silver lining. Dr. Meyer and Brandt met small time swindlers August Wimmers and Gaustave Baum while serving time in jail. The four men became personal friends and planned on combining their devious talents once out of jail. Before they could join forces, Baum was caught on an individual caper and was stashed away in a Cincinnati cooler for two years.

Dr. Meyer had a scheme. He explained to Brandt and Wimmers that using Baum's identity, Brandt would marry Dr. Meyer's cute young wife Marie. A short time after the marriage Baum (even though you and I know he really is Brandt, let's call him Baum from here on in) would purchase life insurance with his every loving wife Marie as the beneficiary. Baum would then be fed poisonous antimony over a prolonged period of time, causing him to become seriously ill. A regular doctor would attend Baum throughout his illness. At the last moment Dr. Meyer would restore Baum to health, substitute a fresh body somewhat similar to Baum in appearance and call in a new doctor. The new doctor would examine the body, and after being urged to consult with the regular attending physician by Marie, he would find out that Baum had been ill and under a physician's care for some months. Under those conditions he should sign the death certificate without hesitation.

Baum married Marie. He then took out $3,500 life insurance with Mutual Life, $3,000 with Washington Life, $1,000 with Aetna, and another $1,000 with New York Life. In all $8,500, a princely sum in the Gay '90s.

Baum, accompanied by Wimmers, moved to New

York City and rented a flat at 320 East 13th St. The first night at supper Wimmers suggested that there was no time like the present to start the poison flowing. Dr. Meyer had provided him with a supply of antimony and suggested that it would be most palatable with a sweet desert. Baum turned chicken. After all, it was fine for everyone to be so enthusiastic, but it was he alone who was to become seriously ill.

The next day Baum again found some lame excuse not to take his poison. Wimmers had no recourse but to call Dr. Meyer and inform him that Baum was behaving like a stubborn child who refused to take his medicine.

Dr. Meyer and Marie whipped over to the Big Apple from Chicago to straighten matters out. Dr. Meyer pleaded, begged, and beseeched Baum to take his poison like a good boy, but nothing worked. Finally Marie assured Baum that she and Dr. Meyer would stay right there in the flat with him to ensure that nothing went wrong.

Each evening Baum was given small doses of antimony. He became unpleasantly ill. Young Dr. S.B. Minden, who had a general practice nearby, was picked to be the attending physician. Dr. Minden was mildly puzzled by Baum's condition. He prescribed some medicine or other and left with the warning that if the patient should become worse, Wimmers should call him again. As the weeks drifted into months, Dr. Minden made several visits to Baum, whom the doctor now considered to be chronically ill.

Baum was going through hell. He felt that the time had come for him to get well and have a nice fresh body take his place. Dr. Meyer assured him that as soon as the time was ripe, he would run down to the morgue, identify some young stiff as his long lost cousin and claim the body. We will never know if Dr. Meyer ever even entertained the thought of substituting a body for Baum. What we do know is that on March 26, 1892, Baum was given a massive dose of arsenic and died in Dr. Meyer's arms. There was no need to find a substitute body now. Baum's would do nicely.

Dr. Minden was called immediately. His patient was dead and duly buried without incident, if you choose to ignore the wailing and carrying on of the spurious Mrs. Baum at graveside. Marie put on quite a show, particularly as she was several months pregnant with what everyone thought was her dead husband's child. Of course we know it was the child of that devil, Dr. Meyer.

The grieving widow went around to the insurance companies and collected the gang's ill gotten gains. Meyers, Wimmers, and Marie set up housekeeping in Toledo. They took in a rather dull, good-looking young girl named Mary Neiss while Marie awaited the blessed event. It wasn't long before Dr. Meyer wanted to pull off the insurance fraud once again. He cautiously approached Mary, who thought it was a great idea. This time the doctor explained that he would become Dr. Hugo Wayler. Mary would be Mrs. Wayler, and would be fed the poison.

It is conceivable that Meyer might have pulled off the entire scheme successfully for the second time, had it not been for the intervention of true love. What the doctor didn't know was that August Wimmers and Mary Neiss were seeing each other on the sly. Wimmers told Mary that the last time the scheme was pulled, Baum died. To make sure that didn't happen to Mary, Wimmers and Mary eloped.

Dr. Meyer was fit to be tied. It was getting so you couldn't trust anyone. As soon as Marie gave birth, the Meyers moved to Detroit in real fear that Wimmers might tell all to the authorities. It took Wimmers a full year, but he did seek out the doctor with blackmail in mind. Finding the medic living in poverty, he dropped the idea. Like Ford, he had a better idea. He went to one of the defrauded insurance companies and made a deal. For $500 he would reveal Dr. Meyer's address. The insurance company took up Wimmers' proposition and that's how Dr. Meyer and the again pregnant Marie were taken into custody.

Marie gave birth to her baby while in jail. The baby died in jail. Marie was never tried for her part in her husband's murderous ways. She died many years later of natural causes.

Dr. Meyer's murder trial began on December 5, 1893, and was a complicated and sensational one in many ways. It was revealed that Baum was alive and well, a fact which caused the prosecution no end of aggravation until they proved that the murder victim was Brandt, posing as Baum.

In the end evil Dr. Meyer was convicted of murder in the second degree and sentenced to life imprisonment. He remained in Sing Sing from 1894 to 1914, a total of 20 years, before being paroled.

DR. J. HERMAN FEIST
1905

It is unusual for a man to stand trial for murder when it is uncertain where and when the crime took place, or if a murder was committed at all. Strange as it first appears, these circumstances did occur back in 1905 in Nashville, Tennessee.

Oscar Mangrum, 35, was the not too bright owner of a barber shop down Nashville way. His wife of nine years, the former Rosa Mason, was an attractive woman of 33 when our little tale of intrigue and possible mayhem took place. The couple had no children.

They had a room and board arrangement at Mrs. Cullom's comfortable establishment on Sixth Ave.

Rosa was quite unlike her husband in many ways. Oscar was an introvert; Rosa had a bubbly, outgoing personality. Where he was content, she was ambitious. To fulfil her energetic nature, Rosa threw herself into working for philanthropic organizations, often heading up charitable fund-raising drives in cities other than Nashville. It was not unusual for Rosa to travel alone to New Orleans, St. Louis and Chicago. She was extremely successful and grew financially independent of her husband. In fact, Rosa sported several diamond rings which were far beyond what the average barber could afford in 1905.

The Mangrums had a friend, their family physician, J. Herman Feist. It was an open secret among their acquaintances that handsome Dr. Feist had more than a professional interest in pretty Rosa. She, in turn, appeared to encourage the attention. Oscar wasn't exactly unaware of what was taking place behind his back. He spoke to Rosa. She seemed to take the matter lightly, but promised to cool it if her friendship with the doctor was a source of embarrassment to her husband.

There matters stood until December 14,1905. For several days Rosa had been planning a business trip to Chicago. She would leave on the 8 p.m. train and arrive in Chicago the next morning. Rosa mentioned to her brother, J.H. Mason, a cashier at the First National Bank, that she had obtained an upper berth for the trip. Her sister, Mrs. Logan Trousdale, thought she was working too hard and should slow down.

It was a Saturday night, a busy one down at the barber shop. Rosa told Oscar it wasn't necessary for him to accompany her to the station. She caught a hack and promised to call him the next day when she arrived at her destination. Oscar was never to see his wife alive again.

When Rosa failed to call him, Oscar phoned the Hotel Newberry in Chicago. His wife had not been there for several months. Distraught and somewhat suspicious, Oscar called his brother-in-law at the bank. He was informed that Rosa had withdrawn her entire savings, the substantial sum of $1,433.62, the day before she left for Chicago. Oscar searched his rooms at Mrs. Cullom's and discovered that Rosa had taken all her jewelry and a trunk of clothing. The thought occurred to him that his wife might have left him for good. Oscar, naturally enough, thought of Dr. Feist, but that worthy gentleman was still in Nashville, attending to his practice as usual.

Weeks passed. Oscar approached Dr. Feist, imploring the doctor to tell him anything he knew about his missing wife. Feist swore he knew nothing. When Rosa's sister spoke to the doctor, she received the same answer.

On January 26, 43 days after Rosa left for Chicago, steamboat pilot George Spence found her body floating in the Ohio River, near Cairo, Ill. Oscar read about the unidentified body in the newspaper and rushed to Cairo. He positively identified his Rosa.

An autopsy served only to add to the mystery. Doctors agreed that the dead woman had been in the water for a lengthy period of time. They could not, however, ascertain when death had occurred, nor could they find the cause of death. The dead woman had not drowned. There were no marks on her body. Her internal organs were healthy.

Had she met with an accident? Had she committed suicide or had she been murdered? If murder had taken place, where was the foul deed committed? The location on the Ohio River, where the body was recovered, was 265 miles from Nashville. Rosa's money and jewels were not found on her body.

The dead woman's movements were traced. The hack driver, who picked her up in Nashville, was located. He swore he dropped her off at the railway station. Rosa's trunk was recovered from the train depot in Chicago, where it had rested since December 15, the day after she disappeared. It seemed that Rosa had checked her trunk and boarded the train for Chicago.

In Nashville, nasty rumors circulated about Dr. Feist's relationship with Rosa. He was seen in Nashville each day in December, but there were those who believed the doctor could have robbed and murdered Rosa at night. Maybe poison was used. The doctor could have thrown Rosa into the river without ever leaving Nashville during daylight hours. Many came forward with information that they had seen Dr. Feist and Rosa in compromising circumstances. It was all only gossip before, but now the relationship took on far more serious connotations.

Based on these innuendoes and rumors, Dr. Feist was arrested and charged with Rosa's murder. His trial was the most sensational to take place in the Southern U.S. in years.

During his trial, evidence was produced indicating that Dr. Feist had never had more than $159 on deposit in his bank at any one time. He had often borrowed money from Rosa. While it was never established what the doctor did with his substantial income, many believed he bet heavily on the horses.

Other doctors occupying the Wilcox Building, where Dr. Feist had his practice, swore that they had seen Rosa and the doctor embrace on several occasions. One had even warned Feist to be more discreet. As the trial progressed, there was little doubt that hanky panky had taken place between the doctor and Rosa, but hanky panky does not a murder case make. There was more.

E.H. Mitchell, a livery stable owner, stated that he received a call from a Dr. S.A. Bean at approximately 8:30 p.m. on December 14. The doctor asked that a rig be delivered to him at the Wilcox Building. Mitchell complied and met Dr. Bean. Next day, he again met Dr. Bean when he picked up his rig, which was mud-splattered inside and out. There was no Dr. Bean listed in Nashville. Mitchell swore that the man he met was Dr. Feist. The defence produced a myriad of witnesses who swore that Mitchell was a habitual liar.

Five passengers had boarded the sleeper car on the night of December 14. Rosa supposedly had Upper 7. Understandably, neither the Pullman conductor nor the porter could remember anything about the passengers. The prosecution insisted that Rosa had checked her trunk through to Chicago, but had not boarded the train. On some ruse or other, Dr. Feist had enticed her into his rented rig and later that night robbed, killed and tossed her into the river. They claimed the body had floated the 265 miles to where it was found.

Defence counsel believed Rosa had boarded the train and, for some reason known only to herself, disembarked at Evansville, Ill. Here she was murdered for her possessions and thrown into the Ohio River, where she was later found.

The presiding judge reminded the jury that there was really no proof that Rosa Mangrum had been murdered. If she had been murdered, there was no proof that the crime had taken place in the jurisdiction in which the trial was being held. Despite these warnings, Dr. Feist was found guilty of murder.

Dr. Feist appealed. It took a full year for the appeal to reach the state Supreme Court. That august body declared that murder had not been proven and reversed the jury's decision. Dr. Feist was not tried again. He immediately left Nashville and never returned.

Was Dr. Feist innocent or guilty? Would a man of his intelligence hire a rig from a man who could later identify him? Very unlikely.

Then again, there are those suspicious souls who relish the convoluted. They claim the wily doctor, deeply in debt, talked Rosa into withdrawing all her money. He had her pack her clothing on the pretence that they were running away together. She purchased a single ticket. To allay suspicion, he told her he would buy his own ticket. At the last minute, after the trunk was checked, he talked her out of taking the train. He then killed her and submerged her body on one of the rivers around Nashville. The doctor had over a month and a half to lug the body the 265 miles to where it was found.

Of course, we will never know whether Dr. Feist was guilty or not. He died without telling a soul.

DR. WALTER WILKINS
1906

Husbands who hasten the departure of their wives should exhibit some sign of physical or emotional anguish. Wailing at the moon, uncontrollable flailing, or even simple tears are recommended. Never, but never, nonchalantly decide to take the dog for a walk. Strangely enough, Dr. Walter Keene Wilkins of Long Beach, N.Y. did just that.

Dr. Wilkins was a kindly appearing gentleman, who sported a fine display of muttonchop whiskers, as was the fashion in 1906. At 67 years of age, he was somewhat older than his dear wife Julia.

One chilly February evening the police of tiny Long Beach received a call from Max Mayer, a neighbor of the Wilkins'. Upon investigating the call, they found Dr. Wilkins bending over his wife's prostrate form in front of their home. He was washing blood from Julia's horribly battered face. The poor woman was rushed to the hospital by ambulance, where two hours later she died. It took some effort to notify the distraught husband. He was busy walking the two family dogs who, incidentally, answered to the rather prosaic names of Duke and Duchess. I might add, but only in passing, that the Wilkins owned a parrot and a monkey, whose names fortunately have been lost to posterity.

Dr. Wilkins had quite a story to tell. He and his wife arrived home from shopping. As they approached their house on Olive St., the doctor thought there was someone inside. He entered alone, advising his wife to stay outside. Suddenly, he was struck a vicious blow to the head.

Luckily, he was wearing a derby hat at the time, which no doubt cushioned the blow. Nonetheless, he was jumped upon by at least three men, but managed somehow to scream a warning to his wife, who in turn yelled for help.

One of the doctor's attackers dashed past his fallen form and obviously hit Julia repeatedly over the head until she lay dying on the sidewalk. Slowly the doctor regained consciousness. He ran to his neighbor's home and raised the alarm. Then he returned to help his wife as best he could.

Robbery had obviously been the motive. The doctor had been robbed of his wallet and diamond stickpin. The house had been ransacked as well. It appeared that three assailants had taken part in the attack. Three glasses and a bottle of the doctor's good brandy were found on the kitchen table. It appeared as if three men were having a drink when the doctor entered the house.

Outside in the yard, the police found a half-inch lead pipe wrapped in cloth. It was surmised that this was the weapon used on Dr. Wilkins. A broken machinist's hammer, held together with wire and wrapped in newspaper, was found beside the unfortunate Mrs. Wilkins.

Now, all of this business of hammers and pipes caused a tremendous amount of excitement around the tiny community of Long Beach. A great deal of pressure was put on the police to come up with the killer. Despite what appeared to be a galaxy of clues, the authorities were hard put to produce a bona fide suspect. In a kind of desperation born of frustration, they decided to look into the benevolent Dr. Wilkins' past. Well, folks, they found out a thing or two.

At the relatively tender age of 35, Wilkins had married one Miss Grace Mansfield. Now Grace wasn't a knockout, but she did have a father who indulged his new son-in-law to the extent of an allowance of $150 a month. When Wilkins failed to make any attempt to support

Mrs. W., she divorced him and returned to being just plain Grace.

In 1893, Dr. Wilkins again entered the holy state of matrimony. This time he wed Suzanne Kirkland, a widow who owned a few rooming houses. The new Mrs. Wilkins fell downstairs one day. During her convalescence from this unfortunate accident she became depressed and nervous. The doctor prescribed ice cold baths. In fact, he filled the tub with ice. Suzanne stepped in and dropped dead. There was no question about it; Dr. Wilkins had a poor track record when it came to wives.

The most recent Mrs. Wilkins had managed to stay married and alive for a full 13 years, but disturbing facts were fast coming to light. Julia had also been married before and had about $100,000 in her name. Dr. Wilkins, it appears, had a fat zero in his name. So much for motive.

The string which had been used to tie newspaper around the murder weapon was traced to a butcher shop where the doctor had purchased the family meat for years. The wire used to repair the mechanic's hammer came from a roll of wire found in the Wilkins' home. It became downright embarrassing when Julia's false teeth were found in the house after the doctor had stated explicitly that his wife never entered the house on the evening she was killed. When it was discovered that the doctor had taken a bloodstained suit to a dry cleaning establishment on the day after the murder, it was just too much. He was arrested and charged.

On June 5, Dr. Wilkins' murder trial began. It immediately became apparent that the evidence against him was overwhelming. When it was revealed that his diamond stickpin, supposedly taken during the course of the robbery, was found in his overcoat, his goose, so to speak, was cooked. The good doctor was found guilty.

The day after the verdict was delivered, Dr. Wilkins

managed to hang himself with a piece of rope from a shower fixture. The doctor, who seemed to have a flair for the dramatic, didn't disappoint, even in death. He left three letters. One provided for Duke, Duchess, the parrot and the monkey. Another revealed that he preferred death to life in Sing Sing, and the third left his lawyer $50 to pay for his cremation.

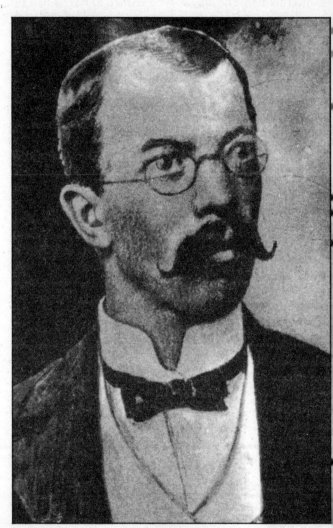

Dr. Hawley Crippen

DR. HAWLEY CRIPPEN
1910

The 35 years between 1875 and 1910 gave rise to a multitude of strange and unusual murders. There were so many people stabbing, strangling and cutting up their fellow men that one hardly knows where to begin. But most of these gentlemen, while they are certainly noteworthy, left their victims where they fell. They didn't experience that blood-chilling confrontation with what has until recently been a fellow human being, and the utterly bothersome task of disposing of the body. So from this era of mass murderers we have plucked a mild, unassuming little man named Dr. Hawley Harvey Crippen.

Hawley was born in Clearwater, Michigan, in 1863, and from the very beginning of his academic career he was considered to be a good student. He was singleminded in his desire to become a doctor, and to this end he studied medicine in Cleveland and New York. After he qualified, he did post-graduate work, becoming an eye and ear specialist. Then he completed his education with further studies in London, England, before returning to the United States, where, between 1885 and 1893, he moved frequently, practising in Detroit, Salt Lake City, New York, St. Louis, Toronto, and Philadelphia.

In 1887, the doctor married one Charlotte Bell, who died, presumably of natural causes, in 1890. After his wife's death, Crippen returned to New York, where he again set up his practice. Dr. Crippen was now a mature 31 years old. He was five feet, seven inches tall, with a decidedly receding hairline, protruding eyes that stared out from behind thick-lensed spectacles, and a small, well-kept moustache. While not altogether a ladies' man, Crippen was neat in appearance and a pleasant, intelligent conversationalist. When he was practising in New York he met a 17-year-old medical secretary called Kunigunde Mackamotzki, who had had the good sense to change her name to Cora Turner. The doctor took one look at Cora's substantial bust, slim waist and well turned ankle and was smitten. The love-struck pair were married almost immediately.

By 1899, the Crippens were living in Philadelphia, and it was here that Cora let the mild Hawley in on a little secret — she wanted to be an opera star. Now, Crippen was no student of voice, but he had heard his wife sing and knew she had a pleasant soprano warble. On occasion, at parties, he would become rather proud when she rendered a tune or two, but an operatic career — that was something else. The little doctor looked quizzically at his wife. Yes, she said, she seriously wanted to study music. Hawley suggested that they relax in the bedroom and continue the discussion about singing another day. No, said Cora, there would be no sex in the Crippen household until she was promised that he would finance her singing lessons. She received a firm promise that very night.

Soon Crippen found that every cent he made was going for singing lessons for his wife. Cora was extremely serious when it came to her career, even to the point of taking the professional name of Belle Elmore. A few years passed, and Cora's singing lessons had practically bankrupted the distraught Crippen. Besides the financial difficulties her singing had brought him, deep down in his heart he didn't think she was all that good.

By 1900, the couple had been husband and wife for eleven years. Like all of us, they had grown older; the doctor was now a worry-racked 42, and his once receding hairline was in full flight, while Cora, at 28, had begun to put on weight and was becoming slovenly in her appearance. More than that, as the months went by, she started to find fault with Hawley. Little by little she had become an overweight nag; and to make matters worse, she had failed to make a name for herself in the singing world. As she became more frustrated with her career, she more and more frequently denied Crippen that which every husband figures is his right. At the Crippen residence, conjugal bliss had given way to continual bickering.

Then the doctor decided to do something about his dilemma. He was offered, and accepted, the position of manager at Munyon's Patent Remedies in London, England. He figured the move would keep him one step ahead of his creditors, as well as providing him and Cora with a welcome change which might improve the climate of their marriage. Cora had other ideas; she felt that at last she would get an opportunity to appear on the stage of the British Music Hall.

The Crippens arrived in London and took furnished rooms in Bloomsbury. Even before they were comfortably settled, Cora started making the rounds of booking agents, trying to get a high-class singing position. She soon lowered her sights, and was satisfied to accept any singing job she could get. But she had one major drawback. While she made placid Hawley buy her expensive clothing to enhance her appearance when auditioning, she simply couldn't sing. She managed to obtain a few engagements in provincial halls, reaching the pinnacle of her career when she appeared on the same bill as George Formby, Sr., at the Dudley New Empire. A short time after this appearance, she was booed off the stage during another performance. Cora was finding out that the road to fame and fortune was a rocky one.

In 1905, the couple moved from Bloomsbury to 39 Hilldrop Crescent in the Holloway district. It was around this time that 22-year-old Ethel Le Neve became Dr.

Crippen's private secretary. The doctor, now in his forties, fell hard for the winsome Ethel, and she for her part was not averse to the positive vibes coming her way from the little doctor. By 1907, Ethel and Hawley were lovers, and not only in the physical sense, for it is a fact that they sincerely loved and cared for each other. Crippen was charmed by the passive, unassuming Ethel, who gave so willingly of herself, in sharp contrast to the domineering, aggressive Cora. And that closed bedroom door in the Crippen residence had to be an additional factor.

Further aggravating an already explosive situation, Cora started to invite her theatrical acquaintances over to Hilldrop Crescent. Cora and her friends hardly missed a day whooping it up, while the mild-mannered doctor would shrug and pay the bills. One day after the gang had left the house, Hawley meekly mentioned to Cora that maybe she should cut down on the expensive food and drink she was serving her friends. Crippen received a blast that could be heard as far away as Stonehenge on a clear day, for even suggesting such a thing. On occasion Cora would do more than party; some evenings she stayed out until the early morning hours, and Crippen knew full well she was having affairs with her broken-down Thespian buddies. On the other hand, Cora was aware that her meek husband was playing around, and if his infidelity managed to keep him out of her hair, so much the better. And so life went on at Hilldrop Crescent, both husband and wife leading separate lives, each tolerating the other's indiscretions.

On January 17, 1910, Dr. Crippen strolled in to Lewis and Burrowes, Chemists, on Oxford Street. He purchased five grains of hyoscin hydrobromide, which, in small doses, is used as a sedative. The clerk had Crippen sign the poisons register — taken in large doses hyoscin hydrobromide is a deadly poison — and remembered the transaction because he could not recall ever having sold such a large amount of the drug before. It can be administered in tea or coffee, and is tasteless. Its effects in massive doses are loss of consciousness, paralysis, and death in a matter of hours.

Two weeks later, on the night of January 31, Cora and Hawley had another couple over for an intimate little dinner party followed by a game of cards. Clara and Paul Martinetti were retired entertainers, who were really friends of Cora's. They had a pleasant enough evening, and left at about one thirty in the morning. The Martinettis were the last people to see Cora alive.

The first sign that all was not normal at the Crippen household came when an organization Cora belonged to — the Music Hall Ladies' Guild — received a letter of resignation advising them that she had to rush to America to take care of a seriously ill relative. The letter was signed by Crippen using his wife's professional name, Belle Elmore, per H.H.C. By word of mouth the news spread that Cora was away in America. Some of her close friends remarked that it was strange that she didn't call someone with an explanation. Still, serious illnesses do strike suddenly and the entertainment set seemed satisfied for the time being.

Then Dr. Crippen commenced to make moves which were not designed to enhance our opinion of his intelligence. He pawned some of Cora's jewelry for £200. On February 12, Ethel Le Neve moved into the house on Hilldrop Crescent, causing tongues to wag. As if that wasn't enough to raise an eyebrow or two, Hawley showed up at a Music Hall Ladies' Ball with Ethel. Only a blind man could have failed to notice that the brooch Ethel was sporting over her left breast was the property of Cora Crippen. Cora's friends didn't like the look of things, and started to ask the doctor embarrassing questions. They simply couldn't get over the idea of Cora leaving without so much as a goodbye. Crippen told the ladies that a relative of his who lived in San Francisco was seriously ill. He had been told that this relative had mentioned him in his will, and as the sum involved was substantial, Cora and he thought that one of them should go to California to protect their interests. He couldn't go due to his workload, so Cora had made the trip. That story pacified the ladies for a few more weeks.

Then the Music Hall Ladies' Guild received a telegram from Dr. Crippen advising them that dear Cora herself was seriously ill in California. An official of the Guild, a Miss Hawthorne, visited Hilldrop Crescent, and found the mild little doctor half crazy with worry. She left the house with tears in her eyes feeling guilty that suspicious thoughts about Crippen should ever have entered her mind.

A few days later Miss Hawthorne received another telegram from Crippen, this time advising her that the worst had happened—Cora had passed away from pneumonia. The ladies of the Guild inquired as to where the funeral would be held; they wanted to send flowers. Dr. Crippen told them that the body was to be cremated and the ashes would be sent back to London. He then inserted a memorial notice in The Era, a theatrical newspaper. Immediately after he placed the notice, he left for a short trip to Dieppe, France. When Cora's friends dropped around to his office, they noticed that Ethel wasn't at her desk. The ladies talked about Ethel's absence for a moment or two, but the consensus of opinion was that it was most natural for Crippen to have given his secretary some time off while he was away.

Ethel, however, had accompanied her lover to France, and was continually at his side, consoling and comforting him. She couldn't help but notice that the doctor carried a large leather hatbox with him when he boarded the boat for the English Channel crossing. When she inquired about the box while in Dieppe, the doctor replied that he had misplaced it during the crossing, and it never entered her mind again.

When the pair returned to London, Crippen found that the suspicions concerning his wife's disappearance had grown. It seems that Mr. Nash, a friend of Cora's, had just returned to London from New York. He had been there while Cora had supposedly passed through the city on her way to California. Nash knew Cora well, and knew how she felt about their mutual friends in New York. He found it incredible that she had never once contacted them. When he told Miss Hawthorne of his suspicions, they decided to contact Scotland Yard.

It was over four months since Cora had last been seen when Chief Inspector Walter Dew and Sergeant Arthur Miller knocked on the door of 39 Hilldrop Crescent. Dr. Crippen amicably invited the officers in for a cup of tea. In a somewhat hesitant manner Inspector Dew broached the reason for their visit. It seems some friends had become suspicious when they noticed Miss Le Neve wearing a piece of jewelry belonging to his wife. Dr. Crippen cleared his throat—there was something he had to explain to the officers—you see, his wife wasn't dead at all; she had run off with a music hall performer named Bruce Miller. She had been "carrying on" with him for some time, and had finally picked up and left without a word to any of her friends. He had been too ashamed and embarrassed to tell anyone the truth, so he had made up the story of his wife's death. In reality, he thought the two lovers had headed for Chicago.

"Now, doctor, about Miss Le Neve and the jewelry?" Crippen didn't bat an eyelash. He explained that his wife had left in such a hurry she had left her jewelry behind. With a knowing wink Crippen admitted that he had taken up with Ethel Le Neve after his wife ran away, and he was now her lover.

The Inspector looked at the sergeant and the sergeant

looked at the inspector. The whole story had a ring of truth to it. The two men conducted a cursory examination of the entire premises and found nothing suspicious. They advised Crippen to place an advertisement in a Chicago paper to assist in finding his wife and still the gossip once and for all. Crippen assured them that he would take their advice. The policemen apologized to Dr. Crippen for the disturbance and returned to the station satisfied that no crime had been committed.

On July 11, 1910, three days after the police visit to Crippen's house, Miss Hawthorne called Inspector Dew for a progress report on the Crippen affair. Dew told Miss Hawthorne that Cora had run away with another man, and that the whole matter was not of concern to the police. Miss Hawthorne informed Dew that something was wrong. Crippen and Le Neve had disappeared. Dew was forced to look into the case again. This time he found out that shortly after his meeting with Crippen on the previous Saturday, July 8, the doctor had written notes to his business associates resigning his position, cleaning out his office, and together with Ethel Le Neve had dropped from sight.

The doctor, who had appeared cool as a cucumber from the first day his wife was noticed to be missing, had finally panicked. Dew questioned Crippen's fellow employees and found a young man who had performed an unusual errand for him. The doctor had asked his colleague to purchase an entire outfit of clothing to fit a boy of sixteen. The young man gave a detailed description of the articles he had purchased for Crippen — brown tweed suit, boots, a hat and an overcoat. After some reflection, Dew came to the conclusion that the clothing had been purchased to disguise Ethel Le Neve in her flight with Crippen. On Tuesday, July 12, Scotland Yard decided to make a thorough search of 39 Hilldrop Crescent. For three days the police peered into and poked at the house while the garden was being dug up. On the third day some loose bricks were discovered under the coal bin in the cellar. The remainder of the floor had mortar between the bricks. The loose bricks were removed, and under a few inches of clay, the police found the remains of Mrs. Crippen — really just "a mass of flesh" wrapped in a pyjama jacket. The body had been dissected and the head was missing.

Inspector Dew checked back on Crippen's actions and found the chemist where he had purchased the hyoscin hydrobromide. Chemical analysis of Cora's remains confirmed that she had met her death as the result of the administration of this drug. On July 16, a warrant was issued for the arrest of Crippen and Le Neve for murder and mutilation. The story was a sensation, and became even more newsworthy because no one seemed to know where to look for the two fugitives. In England, during the time Crippen and Le Neve were at large, little else was discussed. Everyone had a theory about the missing pair, and they were constantly being spotted throughout England and the continent by both the police and the public.

In reality, Dew was on the right track. Crippen had dressed his lover as a boy, and the two of them had left the country, heading for Rotterdam, Holland. The doctor used the alias of John Philo Robinson, and Ethel took on the identity of his son George.

They made their way to Antwerp, Belgium, where on July 20 they booked passage for Quebec City, Canada, on the SS *Montrose*.

It is quite possible that the fugitives would have made good their escape had it not been for the captain of the *Montrose*. Almost from the first hour the pair boarded his ship, the captain noticed the unnatural actions of the Robinsons. He watched the way they held hands, which seemed decidedly odd for a father and son. The second day out of Antwerp he noticed how feminine young Robinson's movements were when he caught a tennis ball on deck. By July 22, the captain was sure that he had Crippen and Le Neve on his ship. Captain Kendall radioed his suspicions to the managing director of the Canadian Pacific Shipping Co. in Liverpool, who passed the message along to Scotland Yard. Several messages went back and forth, and Scotland Yard became convinced that they had located the wanted pair. On July 23, Inspector Dew boarded the *Laurentic*, a much faster ship than the *Montrose*, at Liverpool. It was calculated that Dew would overtake his quarry just before the *Montrose* docked in Canada. The case now took on the aspect of a race. Each day the press carried the relative positions of both ships, vividly illustrating the relentless pursuit of the *Montrose* by the *Laurentic*. The distance between the two ships diminished steadily as the *Montrose* approached Canada.

It is well to remember that the passing of radio messages was relatively new to the public. Guglielmo Marconi had established wireless communication across the Atlantic in 1901. This added feature of the chase captured the imagination, not only of England, but of the entire world. At the time of Crippen's flight for freedom, only about one hundred ships were equipped with radios. Within six months over six hundred ships were so equipped and it is believed the Crippen case was instrumental in making radios a legal requirement for ocean going vessels.

While all this was going on, Crippen and Le Neve thought they had succeeded in evading the authorities, and didn't even know that Cora's body had been discovered. Finally, on July 31 the *Laurentic* caught up with the *Montrose* off Father Point, Quebec. Dew boarded the ship and arranged with Captain Kendall to meet Crippen in the captain's quarters.

"Good morning, Dr. Crippen, I am Chief Inspector Dew."

"Good morning, Mr. Dew," replied Crippen.

"You will be arrested for the murder and mutilation of your wife, Cora Crippen," stated Dew.

"I am not sorry, the anxiety has been too much."

The dramatic confrontation between detective and murderer was over. Extradition proceedings were dispensed with speedily, and the couple were returned to England to stand trial. Crippen's trial took place in October 1910, and took four days to complete. Public interest in the Crippen trial was greater than in any other heard in London's famous Old Bailey. Huge crowds spilled out onto the street. People stood waiting for hours to catch a glimpse of the accused. The proceedings had all the right ingredients —a love triangle, promiscuous relations, poison, a mutilated body, a missing head, drama on the high seas, a beautiful young girl, and a man of medicine gone wrong.

When it was all over Dr. Crippen was found guilty of the murder of his wife. He was executed on the gallows at Pentonville on November 23, 1910. His last request was that a photograph of Ethel be buried with him, and this request was granted and carried out. Crippen went to his death proclaiming Ethel's innocence.

Two weeks after Crippen's trial, Ethel Le Neve stood trial as an accessory after the fact at the Old Bailey. The evidence against her was flimsy, and it is doubtful if she ever realized that she was doing anything more than running away with her lover. Ethel steadfastly professed that she did not even know of Mrs. Crippen's death. She was acquitted, and left for Canada on the day Dr. Crippen was executed.

After five years she returned to England using an assumed name, Ethel Nelson. She married a clerk called Stanley Smith, and lived a quiet life in Croydon, South

London. Only her husband and one other close friend ever knew her real identity. In 1967, 57 years after the Crippen-Le Neve trials, a gentle, grey-haired grandmother, lying close to death in Dulwich hospital, made a last request, that a locket containing a picture of Dr. Hawley Crippen be placed in her casket. So Ethel Le Neve passed from this earth.

DR. ROBERT MacGREGOR
1912

You've already met Canada's most infamous medical murderer, Dr. Neill Cream, who took tremendous delight in poisoning unsuspecting ladies before the turn of the century. Less well known but every bit as wicked was London, Ontario's Dr. Robert MacGregor.

By the time he was 30, Dr. MacGregor had left London and set up practice in the village of Ubly in Huron County, Michigan. One January afternoon in 1909, Carrie Sparling, the 45-year-old wife of dairy farmer John Wesley Sparling, walked into the doctor's office with a distressing bit of dust in her left eye.

Although Carrie was the mother of four strapping sons, she had the appearance of a girl of 25. Dr. MacGregor took one look at the bad eye, coughed and said, "Kindly disrobe." The doctor started by staring at Carrie's toes and after several pauses on his way northward finally concentrated on the sore eye. Dr. MacGregor extracted the dust and told his patient that he would drop in on her the next time he was near her farm in Sanilac County, about an hour's buggy drive from Ubly.

Dr. MacGregor was a tall, attractive man. Carrie didn't exactly repulse his advances. The doctor did have a meek, rather ugly wife of his own, who was forgotten from the very day Carrie showed up with that bad eye.

A week after Carrie's visit, Dr. MacGregor travelled to the Sparling farm, where he met big husky, John Wesley Sparling and his four sons, Ray, 20, Scyrel, 21, Albert, 23, and Peter, 24.

The doctor thought it best to give Carrie a physical

examination. One never knew what damage dust in the eye could inflict. Dr. MacGregor and Carrie were directed to the bedroom by trusting John Wesley. An hour later they emerged and advised Mr. Sparling, "Everything was just fine, even better than we had hoped."

From then on Carrie suffered from a series of minor ailments. The doctor came every second week or so and never failed to cure what ailed her.

After several months had passed, Dr. MacGregor confided to his best friend Xenophon A. Boomhower, who lived in the neighboring village of Bad Axe, that he suspected John Wesley Sparling had Bright's disease. A few months later John Wesley was confined to his bed. Despite Dr. MacGregor's care, the poor man was called to that great dairy farm in the sky.

The doctor, who was now considered a dear family friend by the four boys and something altogether different by Carrie, met with the Sparling family. He advised the boys to take out life insurance. Considering the untimely demise of their father, the four lads thought it good advice. By coincidence, the doctor's father was an insurance agent back in London. He sold them Sun Life of Canada policies.

A year later Dr. MacGregor informed his friend Boomhower that Pete Sparling had acute pancreatitis. Everyone was shocked. Poor Pete. He was laid to rest beside his dad less than a year after the elder Sparling had departed this mortal coil.

Distraught, Carrie decided to sell the farm and purchase a smaller one in Huron County, a stone's throw from Dr. MacGregor's office in Ubly. Coincidental with the Sparlings' move, good friend Xenophon Boomhower was appointed county prosecutor.

The wood was hardly stacked for the winter at the Sparlings' new farm when Albert took ill. The doctor explained to Boomhower that Albert had lifted a heavy piece of farm machinery and had suffered internal injuries. A few months later Albert joined Pete and John Wesley down at the family plot.

It was vacation time. Dr. MacGregor took his wife on a motoring trip throughout Ontario. While the doctor was away, Carrie bought a house in Ubly for investment purposes. It was only a few streets removed from Dr. MacGregor's office. When the MacGregors returned, Carrie suggested that they move out of their present home and rent from her. It seemed like a good idea, and that's how the MacGregors became tenants of Carrie Sparling.

Mrs. MacGregor took ill. Her husband suggested she return to Ontario to visit relatives and rest up. Mrs. MacGregor left the scene. She was no sooner gone than Carrie took to visiting the good doctor. Sometimes she stayed all day. When the fancy struck her she stayed all night. Tongues wagged, but the untimely death of Scyrel Sparling interrupted the gossip.

The death appeared to puzzle Dr. MacGregor. He suggested an autopsy, which he conducted with another doctor in attendance. It was a cursory affair. Dr. MacGregor took one look and said, "Well, well, cancer of the liver." The other doctor agreed without really taking part in the examination. Scyrel joined the other members of his family down at the eternal place of rest.

Shortly after Scyrel's tragic passing, a village busybody observed Carrie leaving the doctor's residence at dawn. She informed elderly John Sparling, an uncle of the late John Wesley, who waited until he spied Carrie enter Dr. MacGregor's home. He then climbed up a ladder and peered into the bedroom. Land sakes! The rumors were true. There were Carrie and Dr. MacGregor, coupled.

Things got hot. Old John informed Prosecutor Boomhower, who secretly had Scyrel's body exhumed. Vital organs were sent to the University of Michigan. The university report stated that Scyrel's organs were laced with arsenic. Albert's body was also exhumed. It, too, contained arsenic.

When Dr. MacGregor told Boomhower that the one remaining Sparling son, Ray, had taken ill, he knew he had to take immediate action. Unknown to Carrie, he visited the bedridden Ray at the farm and told him the whole sordid story. He advised Ray to pretend to take Dr. MacGregor's medicine but to save it for analysis. The medicine proved to be laced with arsenic.

Dr. MacGregor was taken into custody and charged with Scyrel's murder. Carrie was charged with being an accomplice. During the trial, Prosecutor Boomhower forcefully pointed out that both Albert's and Scyrel's bodies had contained arsenic. Dr. MacGregor was found guilty and sentenced to life in Michigan State Prison. The charges against Carrie were dropped.

As soon as the prison gates closed behind him in 1912, Dr. MacGregor began a campaign of letter writing proclaiming his innocence. One such letter reached Gov. Woodbridge Fuller, who was appalled that testimony concerning Albert's poisoning had been admitted as evidence at a trial which concerned Scyrel's death only. The governor interviewed several members of the jury, who said they would not have found MacGregor guilty if the evidence concerning Albert's death had not been presented.

Gov. Fuller pardoned Dr. MacGregor after he had served four years in prison. Once outside, the doctor was the object of ridicule. Friendless, he applied for the position of physician at Michigan State Prison. The appointment was granted. Dr. MacGregor ministered to the prisoners for 12 years, never leaving the institution until he died within its grey walls in 1928.

DR. ARTHUR WAITE
1917

It is seldom in the annals of crime that a man can first be suspected, then arrested and finally stand trial for murder without ever taking the entire matter seriously. One man went through the entire ordeal, laughing and joking to the end.

Dr. Arthur Warren Waite was born in Grand Rapids, Mich. in 1887. He took his dental surgeon's degree in Glasgow, Scotland, and practised in South Africa before returning to the United States at the age of 28. Dr. Waite married Clara Peck, the daughter of a Grand Rapids millionaire in September 1915. Then he set up practice in New York City and at the same time did pure research at the Cornell Medical School. He played a good game of tennis, led an active social life, and all in all appeared to be a man who had everything.

There was one thing though; you see, the doctor decided to kill all his relatives.

Mrs. John E. Peck was Art's mother-in-law. Her daughter and the charming dentist were married for three months when she decided to visit the couple over the Christmas holidays. She arrived a healthy, robust woman. By January 30, she was dead. A doctor certified that she had died of kidney disease.

Art informed Clara that her mother had confided in him during her brief illness that she wished to be cremated. Clara thought it strange that her mother had never mentioned this to her, but gave her consent to the request.

After his wife's funeral, Mr. Peck came to visit with his

daughter and son-in-law. He was dead by March 12. Again, the doctor called it kidney disease and the body was to be cremated. Apparently Mr. Peck had confided this wish to Arthur and no one else. Dr. Art made all the arrangements. He had the body embalmed, and then it was to be shipped to Grand Rapids to allow the rest of the family to pay their last respects. Finally the remains were to be forwarded to Detroit for cremation.

Everything went according to plan, until the party accompanying the body met the rest of the family in Grand Rapids. Here, Clara's brother Percy, who never got along with Art, acted very hostile to the dentist. He had received an anonymous letter telling him not to allow his father's body to be cremated. Percy decided to take over all the details concerning his father's body. Arthur and Clara returned to New York.

Meanwhile, Percy gave the order to have an autopsy performed on his father. Then at his urging the authorities started to look more closely into Arthur's background. They found that as a student, Arthur had stolen money, and later in South Africa had tried to marry a wealthy lady whose father had him chased out of the country. Then the story broke that charming, considerate Art was having an affair with a married singer named Margaret Horton. We begrudgingly have to give him a certain amount of credit. It isn't easy to get married, kill your mother-in-law and father-in-law, and carry on with a mistress, all within a period of five months.

The floss that broke the dentist's drill was when five grains of arsenic were found in Mr. Peck's body. This was too much even for Art; he took some poison and when the police went to arrest him, they found him almost dead. He survived and stood trial for double murder.

It was during the trial that Dr. Waite distinguished himself. For starters, despite pleading not guilty, he never once denied killing his in-laws. In fact, he described the whole thing in detail. He even cracked jokes to the jury while he recounted the sordid affair.

In his own words, he said: "I started poisoning her from the very first meal after she arrived. I gave her six assorted tubes of pneumonia, diphtheria and influenza germs in her food. When she finally became ill and took to her bed, I ground up 12 five-grain Veronal and gave her that, too, last thing at night." Art woke up in the middle of the night, found his mother-in-law dead, and went back to sleep. He had ready access to the germs from his research work at the medical school.

Art went on to tell how Mr. Peck didn't die easy. He tried several types of poisons on him, but nothing seemed to work. He went through his supply of germs, then tried chloroform, and finally in desperation he held a pillow over his father-in-law's nose and mouth until he was dead.

The obliging dentist volunteered that he tried to kill his wife's aunt, Catherine Peck, by giving her ground glass in her food when she had visited at Christmas. He only spared her because he switched his attention to his mother-in-law, who seemed to be easier to finish.

In his jocular way the dentist explained that, if he had more time, he would have also poisoned his wife. Art thought this so humorous that he laughed out loud while giving his statement from the witness stand.

He wasn't all fun and games. It was learned that behind the scenes he had attempted to bribe two members of the jury. He also had paid an embalmer to put arsenic in an embalming fluid sampler, so that when the police tested it they would find arsenic, thereby explaining its presence in Mr. Peck's body.

The doctor said his motive for the double murder was to inherit his in-laws' fortune. He even joked that he had done his wife a favor by speeding up her inheritance. His mistress, Margaret Horton, testified that Arthur actually told her that he killed his wife's parents. He said he planned on going to an asylum for a short time as an imbecile.

Dr. Waite was found guilty. He carried off his charade to the bitter end, requesting that he be put to death at the earliest possible date. On May 24, 1917 he arose, ate a hearty breakfast and read a book of John Keats' poems. He then joked with his guards as he walked calmly into the execution chamber and was put to death in the electric chair.

DR. WILMER HADLEY
1918

Wilmer Amos Hadley pursued religion, medicine and members of the opposite sex with unequal vigor. He was always partial to women.

Wilmer was a good ol' boy from Friendswood, Texas. At 20 years of age, he heeded the call, venturing to Wichita, Kansas to study theology. Wilmer's ecclesiastical career lasted two years. One night he ventured into the town's small but active red light district, where he discovered the joys of the flesh. He dropped the religious game like a hot potato. Instead, he took up with a local belle, Bertha Lollar, and ended up marrying the girl.

Now divested of any clerical restraints, Wilmer went home with his new wife. He finagled a job in his father's large dry goods store, but found the cloth of his dad's store no more fulfilling than the cloth of his previous calling. He decided to take up the noble profession of medicine. To further this pursuit, he enrolled in Galveston State University.

Bertha, staunch lass that she was, took a job in order to help pay the cost of her husband's education. She even found time to present him with a bouncing baby boy.

On June 2, 1911, our Wilmer graduated with honors. He divorced Bertha and started his new life by hanging up his shingle in the town of Dickinson, Texas.

It didn't take long for Wilmer to have the largest practice in town. Not only was he a better than average sawbones, he also had an extremely soothing bedside manner with women. Those ladies who were disappointed with their work-weary husbands' performance, were invigorated and thrilled to consent to the doctor's unique treatment.

Dr. Hadley appeared to have everything — a thriving practice, the respect of his neighbors, and a bevy of local beauties more than willing to share his bed. But the good doctor wanted wealth — I mean real wealth. He looked around and homed in on the millionaires from Dallas and Galveston who spent their summer months on ranches near Dickinson.

One fine day the gods smiled down on lascivious Wilmer. He was asked to minister to a young morsel named Sue Kathleen Tinsley, the guest of Commodore E.M. Hartrick. Sue had a bad sunburn. She also had everything else in all the right places. The doctor cultivated the romance and reaped the harvest.

On October 13, 1913, Wilmer and Sue were married. Sue's sister paid for the shindig, which sort of surprised Wilmer. When he questioned his new bride, he discovered for the first time that her once rich daddy had lost his entire fortune. Wilmer flipped, but there was very little he could do other than bide his time. Demonstrating the patience of Job, the man of medicine kept his eyes open for his next try at the brass ring.

Wilmer figured that Colorado, with its wealthy silver miners, should be ripe for picking. Besides, the miners' wives should be sufficiently neglected to be susceptible to a large dose of his particular cure-all. Wilmer and Sue settled in Eagle County. The doctor had figured correctly. He soon owned a thriving private hospital, chock-full of women with an assortment of minor ailments and some with no ailments at all. It didn't matter to Wilmer. He cured what ailed each and every one.

Rumors of the doctor's peccadilloes spread throughout the county. A few robust silver millionaires got together with the idea that the district would be a far better place without the virile doctor. Wilmer didn't have to be told twice. He sold the hospital and headed for Red Cliff, Colo., where he was hired to run a hospital owned by Empire Zinc. The job came with the usual perks for Wilmer — nurses.

But a man of Wilmer's greed can only live on love for a limited period of time. He still wanted a wealthy wife. Maybe doctoring in the service would put him in touch with a rich Southern belle. Wilmer joined the army and was assigned to Debarkation Hospital No. 52 at Westhampton, Virginia.

As luck would have it, he met nurse Cheryl Johnson, who was everything a red-blooded southern peach should be, without the pit. This time, Wilmer didn't take any chances. He consulted Dun and Bradstreet. Sure enough, Cheryl's daddy was a financial heavyweight. Wilmer commenced his campaign with the flair of a Patton and the attention to detail of an Eisenhower. It only took three dates before Cheryl was enjoying the doctor's physical attributes. There was talk of marriage. Serious talk. Daddy and Mummy Johnson consented.

Almost forgotten was everloving wife Sue. Cheryl knew that her true love was married, but firmly believed that Sue was in California finalizing her divorce. Nothing could be further from the truth. At this crucial juncture in his campaign, Wilmer received a call from Richmond. Sue was on her way for a visit. Wilmer did a neat bit of footwork. He rented a furnished room, met and made passionate love to his wife, and then formulated intricate plans to kill her.

It was a momentous day, November 11, 1918, the day the armistice was signed ending World War I. Wilmer took Sue for a boat ride on the James River. He brought along a bottle of whisky, liberally laced with a drug which would render his wife unconscious. Once this was accomplished, it would be a simple matter to dump her overboard. A tragic accident, a drowning. Why, Wilmer could see the headlines: Doctor Makes Heroic Attempt to Save Wife.

He offered Sue a drink. It was cold that November afternoon out on the river. Sue took a healthy gulp, swayed and keeled over. Wilmer was just about to dump her overboard when he absently felt for a pulse, as doctors sometimes do. He was shocked. Sue was dead. As any fan of Agatha knows, if a person is dead before being submerged in water, there will be no water in the lungs. That's a prerequisite to drowning. Wilmer had to improvise. He tied Sue up with a rope and the boat's anchor. Then he dropped the whole bundle overboard.

Wilmer went ashore and faked checking his wife out of the furnished room, explaining that she was moving into larger quarters with him. He packed her belongings in a trunk, which he shipped to Atlanta, to be held there until he called.

Details, details — they were cumbersome. But in a few hours they were completed, enabling the murderous doctor to keep his date with wealthy Cheryl that very night.

A few days later, Wilmer wrote to Sue's sister, advising her that Sue had become seriously ill on a cruise to Puerto Rico. Unfortunately, she had died of natural causes. It had been tragic.

On December 5, Dr. Hadley received his discharge from the army. He told Cheryl he had to travel to Texas to prepare their new home and make arrangements to practise there. Cunning Wilmer travelled via Atlanta, where he picked up Sue's trunk. While he was in Atlanta, Sue's body was discovered, caught in some bushes at the edge of the James River.

It was a month and a half after the murder and the body was badly decomposed. However, the woman who had rented the furnished room to Dr. Hadley, identified some of the clothing found on the body as belonging to Mrs. Hadley. Sue's sister was called in. She identified her sister's ring. The hunt for the missing husband had just started when the coroner announced that Sue Hadley was a possible murder victim.

Wilmer felt the heat. He stayed one step ahead of the law for two years before being tracked down by Pinkerton detectives in August 1921. He was bedded down with two young Mexican girls in San Juan County, New Mexico when he was taken into custody.

Brought back to Richmond, Wilmer confessed to killing Sue. He added the little white lie that she was having an affair with one of his friends. His story didn't hold much water. At the time the friend was accused of having the affair, he was serving overseas in France with the armed forces.

Wilmer was tried and found guilty of his wife's murder. On October 27, 1921, Dr. Wilmer Hadley was executed in the electric chair in Richmond, Va.

DR. THOMAS YOUNG
1925

It is difficult to apprehend a murderer when no crime is known to have been committed.

Grace Hunt hailed from a well-known California family. When she met and married Patrick Grogan in 1909, her happiness seemed assured. After all, Pat Grogan had made a fortune in the olive trade and was a bona fide millionaire. Grace and Pat had one son, Charles.

As the years drifted by, Grace and her husband agreed to disagree. When Charles was 10, she and Patrick were divorced. The divorce was a civilized affair. Grace was given custody of Charles and a cool half million dollars to soothe any hurts and to keep the wolf from the door.

There were wolves of a far different kind at Grace's door. She was an attractive young woman with oodles of cash, just waiting for the right swain to come a-calling.

Two years later, when Patrick died, leaving the balance of his estate to his son, with Grace sole administratrix, she became an extremely attractive catch indeed. After Patrick had been duly planted, Grace became a regular in Los Angeles' social circles. Many a young stud with one eye on Grace's figure and the other on the figures in her bank book courted the widow with a vengeance. One such suitor emerged with the prize.

Dr. Thomas Young was a newly turned out dentist who had decided to establish his practice among the socially prominent of Los Angeles. He fixed his sights on Grace like the lead hound pursuing the fox. Initially, Grace rejected the dentist, but eventually his persistence paid off.

In the winter of 1923, Grace became Mrs. Thomas Young. For two years, Dr. Young's practice flourished, as did his marriage to Grace. The attractive couple were seen in the best restaurants and were asked to the most prestigious parties. The Youngs were definitely leading the good life in Lotusland.

And then it happened. On February 22, 1925, Dr. Young contacted Los Angeles police, informing them that his wife Grace had disappeared. The dentist told his story.

Twenty-four hours earlier, he and Grace had left their Beverley Glen cottage for dinner in Venice. They had a few drinks, enjoyed dinner and were about to leave the restaurant when they happened to bump into a woman he knew. It was nothing more than a chance meeting, but afterwards Grace flew into a jealous rage. According to Young, this was not an isolated incident. Grace was insanely jealous. Embarrassed, he hustled his wife out to their car.

While driving back to Los Angeles, Grace was beside herself with rage. During the trip, she took a swing at her husband and broke his glasses. Eventually, she quieted down and even apologized for causing a scene. The Youngs made up and decided to drop into Los Angeles' Hotel Biltmore to dance and have a few drinks.

Grace excused herself in the lobby of the hotel and made her way to the powder room. As far as her husband knew, no one had seen her since that moment. Dr. Young added that Grace was carrying $150,000 in negotiable securities and all her jewelry. In total, Grace was lugging around a quarter of a million dollars on her person. Young's statement begged the question — why would a woman carry a fortune in her purse? Dr. Young told police he thought his wife may have been afraid that their cottage in Beverley Glen was susceptible to being burglarized.

The unusual disappearance made front page headlines.

It's not often that a socially prominent woman disappears carrying a fortune in her purse.

A few weeks after the disappearance, Grace's friends began to receive letters, apparently in Grace's handwriting. The letters were postmarked from towns and cities within 500 miles of Los Angeles. In these letters, Grace informed friends that she was tired of the incessant arguments with her husband. She planned to get away from it all for a while in Europe.

It all seemed so perfect, except for one thing. Anyone who knew Grace realized that she would write or contact her son, Charles, if she were leaving her home for any prolonged period of time. Grace's father, Earl R. Hunt, was not satisfied with the way the investigation was being conducted. He hired the famed Burns Detective Agency to find out what had happened to his daughter. Dr. Young hired another detective agency to locate his wife. In all, there were now three different organizations searching for Grace Young.

Months passed. The investigation wound down. Dr. Young and Charles spent a lot of time together at their cottage. Gradually, Young started to live a normal life again. He even threw a few parties for friends.

Early that summer, the Burns Detective Agency came up with the disconcerting information that Dr. Young's secretary had been seen wearing one of Grace's rings. When questioned, the secretary said Young had showed up at work one day with the ring. She had worn it for a day or so and had returned it to him. For the first time, it was discovered that Dr. Young had lied. He had told police that his wife had taken all her jewelry with her. The Burns boys shared their information with the authorities.

A meeting was held. It was decided that the various organizations conducting inquiries into Grace Young's disappearance share their information. It seems everyone had found out something which incriminated Dr. Young.

Since his mother's disappearance, Charles Grogan had changed his will, which had previously left everything to his mother. His new will made his stepfather sole beneficiary.

Witnesses were located who swore Grace had been carrying a tiny purse on the night she disappeared. It could not possibly have held all her jewelry as well as negotiable securities. The Burns Agency had unearthed the hitherto unknown fact that Young had been married twice before.

Police were successful in obtaining a search warrant to go over the Beverley Glen cottage during Young's absence. They found a three carat diamond ring.

Dr. Young was questioned. When he was shown the ring, he was as cool as a cucumber, claiming that Grace often placed various pieces of her jewelry in the side pockets of their automobile. He had found the ring in the car and had placed it with his personal papers in the cottage. Dr. Young apologized for not informing police that he had found the ring.

Everyone concerned was now sure that Young was lying, but they had absolutely no proof that he had committed any crime. In fact, they had no positive proof that any crime had been committed at all.

On June 14, 1925, Young was brought to police headquarters for another round of questioning. Worn to a frazzle by the constant harassment, he broke down and revealed what had happened to Grace. He blurted out that she had accidentally struck her head and had fallen into a cistern at their cottage.

Police rushed out to the cottage. In the cistern, under a thin layer of concrete, they uncovered the body of Grace Young. A piece of rubber tubing was in her mouth. Dr. Young changed his story. He now told police that after an argument in the hotel, he had taken his wife to his office, where he had given her enough Scotch to render her unconscious. He then drove to the cottage and put her to bed. He administered a gas called sommonoform (used by dentists during that era) through a rubber tube until Grace was dead. Then he threw her body into the cistern.

The very next day, he had Charles mix the cement which was to cover Grace's body. Young told police, "I had covered the body with newspapers and I thought it would be a great joke on the boy to have him unknowingly cover his mother's body with cement."

Dr. Young went on to state that he had killed Grace to get rid of her and obtain her fortune. He revealed that he was planning to kill his stepson Charles and place him in the cistern as well.

Dr. Young's murder trial was in its tenth day when he was found dead in his cell. He had managed to strangle himself with a piece of wire.

DR. HERMAN SCHMITZ
1926

Sending human parts through the mail is definitely in poor taste. In Canada, our criminals rarely use Canada Post, no doubt firmly believing that any alternate mode of delivery would be less tardy. Not so in Europe, where the mails have often been used to advantage.

On April Fool's Day of 1926, the chief of police of Vienna, Herr Weitzel, was somewhat taken aback when he opened a personally addressed small package which had arrived by mail. It contained a human finger.

The chief turned the distinctive digit over to his lab. No sooner had he finished his strudel break than the lab boys provided him with a full report. The finger was the first finger from a woman's right hand. It was slender, the nail being well manicured and polished. The finger was free of calluses and was quite possibly that of a middle-aged woman. It had been recently severed with surgical skill.

The string and paper used to wrap the package were in common use and proved impossible to trace. The parcel had been mailed in Vienna.

Weitzel rubbed his goatee and thought of the possibilities. Of course, the distasteful parcel could be the prank of a medical student or mortuary employee, but the chief couldn't take a chance. He had to assume a crime had been committed.

While the Vienna police were checking out missing persons and calling on mortuaries, Weitzel received another parcel. You guessed it, the package contained another human finger. It was the third finger from the same hand which had provided the previous finger. Examination of the nail indicated that it was polished with the same nail polish. Medical examination revealed a rather disconcerting fact. The finger had been amputated with surgical skill while the victim was alive.

A plain gold ring was on the finger when it arrived. The ring was made of 22 carat gold. Tiny scratches or indentations on the underside of the ring had been made by the corrosive action of a diluted acid. The acid had many commercial uses, but the one detectives homed in on was its use in the removal of tattoos.

In order to find out if the amputated finger had ever been tattooed, it was necessary to remove the top skin. Once this was done, doctors were able to make out the image of a snake wound around the finger in the exact location covered by the gold ring. There was little doubt in the minds of the investigators that the acid used to remove the tattoo had made the indentations in the ring. But what did it all mean? Maybe the snake held some significance at one time, but had been displaced by the ring.

Tattoo parlors were canvassed, but police were unsuccessful in locating the one where the snake had been applied and removed. The ring also proved impossible to trace.

The story was leaked to the press, which caused Vienna police no end of embarrassment. Was a killer on the loose who took great relish in taunting the entire police force? Above all, could the chief expect further fingers to show up in his mail?

A week passed. The mystery deepened when a female body sans head and two fingers from the right hand was found in a swamp outside Vienna. An examination of the torso shed no light on the identity of the middle-aged victim. However, it was noted that the two fingers had been removed with skill and the use of surgical instruments.

Police were able to make a plaster cast of a footprint

found in soft mud near the torso. From the footprint, an anthropologist gave a description of the man who had made it. It was ascertained that he was over six feet tall, with broad shoulders and long arms.

Weitzel and his boys now had something to work with. They were looking for a tall doctor, most likely a surgeon. They came up with several in Vienna, but gradually all were eliminated. All except one.

Dr. Herman Schmitz was a surgeon who had a small practice, catering mainly to wealthy patients. A search of criminal records revealed that at one time Dr. Schmitz had been charged with malpractice, but had been found innocent by a jury. Despite the verdict, the doctor's practice had suffered. Eventually he gravitated to a small but lucrative practice. His patients obviously were unaware of his past.

A cursory investigation of Schmitz's family revealed that he had a wife and children. The children were of school age and Frau Schmitz seemed happy enough. That's what a cursory investigation indicated. An in-depth investigation uncovered the mistress. It was somewhat of a disappointment for the Vienna detectives to find out that she was alive and well. The victim had to be someone else.

Twenty-four-hour surveillance teams were put on the good doctor, the dear wife and the willing mistress. The doctor stayed clean. So did the wife. But the mistress unwittingly led police to paydirt.

Detectives found a dress shop where the doctor's mistress had a charge account. In those long ago days before credit cards, kept ladies had their bills forwarded to their gentlemen friends every month or so. Vienna police, now hot to trot, questioned the store manager. He told them that the doctor's current mistress was somewhat of a pain, unlike his previous mistress, Anna Stein. He explained that Anna had purchased far more dresses before the doctor had changed horses in midstream.

Police dashed over to Anna's apartment only to find that she had vacated the premises three weeks earlier. A survey of her regular haunts brought the same results. Anna Stein had disappeared. Police were pretty sure they knew the location of her torso and two fingers. However, they weren't sure about her head.

This puzzle was solved when they surreptitiously searched Dr. Schmitz's office. The found a small laboratory off the main office. There, reposing in a bucket of preservative solution was the head of Anna Stein. Dr. Schmitz was picked up and charged with the murder of his mistress.

A meticulous search of the doctor's office turned up pieces of Anna's clothing, which had been partially burned. The doctor's current mistress was somewhat distressed to discover that several pieces of jewelry which had been given to her by Schmitz had once belonged to the deceased.

Witnesses were located who stated that Anna had been furious with her lover when she found out she had been replaced in his affections by a younger woman. They had argued fiercely, but the charming doctor sweet talked Anna into bringing her belongings to his office under the pretence of taking a long holiday in Paris. Anna fell for the ruse. Instead of a trip to the City of Light, she was first made helpless by dope, had two fingers amputated and was then murdered.

Dr. Schmitz admitted to quarreling with his former mistress, but claimed she had thrown herself upon him and expired as a result of a heart attack. Examination of the body proved beyond a doubt that Anna had not died of a heart attack. She had been administered a lethal injection of potassium cyanide. Police found a bottle of diluted acid used to remove the tattooed snake from the dead woman's finger. This had been done to hamper identification of the victim.

Dr. Schmitz's trial for murder promised to be a sensation. The Austrian press carried little else on its front pages. But the drama of a sensational murder trial was not to be. Dr. Schmitz attempted to escape from jail. He made his way to the roof of the building and tried to jump to an adjoining lower roof. He didn't make it. He died on the ground after confessing to the murder of Anna Stein.

Why did the doctor send those fingers to the chief of police? It is believed he never forgave police for their investigation of the malpractice charge brought against him years earlier. He sent the fingers through the mail in an attempt to make the police appear foolish and incompetent. Instead, he drew attention to himself, which eventually caused his death.

DR. THOMAS DREHER
1927

Come on down Louisiana way to swamp land, where Cajuns still love to pot 'gators and wash down their jambalaya with a good swig of rotgut bourbon. That's where Ada and Jim Le Boeuf were born, lived, and died.

Ada, an attractive southern girl, was only 18 when she married Jim in 1907. A big, gruff, quiet man, Jim was easily brought to the boiling point. No one messed around with Jim Le Boeuf. Ada liked that quality, which brought respect from other men. She would eventually grow to fear it.

Jim, who had little formal education, started out as a laborer, but ended up as the manager of the Morgan City Power Plant. For a man with his limited ability, he did rather well for himself. He and Ada had a fine home in Morgan City, their own automobile, life insurance, and four children.

On the surface their marriage appeared to be loving and stable. Below this veneer lay the seeds of discontent. As each year went by Ada slipped further and further into drudgery. She washed, she cleaned, she cooked. She was a good mother, a good wife. But she was still a young woman and desperately longed for something better.

The gruff male quality she had so admired in Jim gradually became boring and even despised. Jim was extremely jealous and his constant suspicions only added to Ada's dislike of her husband and her life. In short, Ada was in a rut. Jim's life was in direct contrast to Ada's. He loved to hunt and fish and spent all his spare time at these activities. Sometimes he would be gone for days with his closest friend, Dr. Thomas E. Dreher and the doctor's rather crude friend, Jim Beadle.

Dr. Dreher had established his practice over 25 years before and was one of the town's leading citizens. He was a married man, with a son studying medicine at Tulane University. A good doctor, Dreher never pressed his patients for payment and often accepted whatever they could afford. Everyone in town loved Dr. Dreher.

Now and then someone might remark that Jim Beadle didn't appear to be a suitable companion for the doctor, but others realized Beadle was an expert shot and there was no one better at handling a small boat. The doctor paid Jim Beadle for his services as a loyal guide.

Morgan City had little to offer the bored Ada Le Boeuf in the way of diversion. Perhaps it was inevitable that she and her husband's best friend, Dr. Dreher, would get together. The opportunities were plentiful. Dreher was the Le Boeufs' family physician. He often visited their home socially and professionally. Ada and the doctor became lovers.

As the years passed there were many in the close-knit community who knew very well that Dr. Dreher was bedding down with his best friend's wife. Of course, Jim Le Boeuf had no idea of his wife's infidelity until someone sent a note to Mrs. Dreher. Poor, timid Mrs. Dreher, who really doesn't enter our story as anything other than a victim of circumstances, paid a visit to Jim Le Boeuf.

Jim saw red. While he couldn't prove the serious accusations that Ada vehemently denied, he managed to make his wife's life miserable. Jim swore that if he ever got even a smidgen of proof, he would kill both his best friend and his wife. Ada didn't doubt it for a minute. Jim didn't go fishing or hunting with the doctor and Jim Beadle any more.

In 1927 the Mississippi overflowed its banks, resulting in one of the worst floods on record. Morgan City was hard hit. Only two streets escaped the flood waters. Still, the citizens of Morgan City were accustomed to coping with floods. Soon their boats could be seen darting up one street and down another. Life went on.

Naturally, with Jim's strong suspicions, coupled with the flood, Ada's and Dr. Dreher's opportunities for romance diminished. Ada had one confidante, a Mrs. Noah Hebert, who could be trusted to deliver messages to the doctor.

On July 1, 1927, Ada sent her lover a message. It read: "Jim and me will go boat riding on the lake tonight. I talked to him and I believe he will treat you friendly. So meet me tonight and fix this up friendly and we will be friends. I am tired of living this way hearing Jim say he is going to kill both of us. As ever, Ada."

The note sounds almost innocent, but later there were those who claimed that the language was purposely guarded and that the note was in reality Jim Le Boeuf's death warrant. That night Dr. Dreher and his friend, Jim Beadle, stepped into their green pirogue, a canoe-like boat, and paddled silently into the night.

Ada and Jim hitched two boats to their car and drove over to Ada's sister's home for supper. They would go for a boat ride after they dined. It was a beautiful night. When they went boating the Le Boeufs always used two boats. Ada was an excellent oarswoman.

After supper the pirogues were taken down from the car. Ada's sister's home was almost surrounded by flood waters. The two boats were launched into a nearby street. Ada suggested they row over a route known to them both, which would lead to Lake Palourde.

The pirogues made their way into the dark night. Slowly houses disappeared from view. The muddy swamp water glistened in the moonlight. The trees hung heavy with Spanish moss. Wild flowers peeked out from the decayed branches of long dead trees. It was a night made for murder. Ada carefully led her husband to his death.

The Le Boeufs paddled silently. Gradually they discerned the outline of two men in a boat directly in their path. One of the men shouted, "Is that you, Jim?" "Yes, who's that?" Jim replied.

A shotgun flashed twice, the noise of the reports roaring across the water. Ada turned quickly and rowed away. Jim Le Boeuf would torment her no more. He lay dead in his boat.

Quickly, two 65-pound railway angle irons were tied to the body. A knife glistened and in an instant the dead man's stomach was slit open. The body was dumped overboard, the boat sunk, and the two shadowy figures rowed away.

Next morning Ada told her children that she and their father had had a terrible quarrel the night before and he had left. No doubt he would be back when he cooled off.

Six days later some men were hunting alligators on Lake Palourde. They found Jim Le Boeuf's body lying face down under a few inches of water. The heavily weighted body had been prevented from sinking by a small submerged tree.

Ada immediately came under suspicion. She was questioned for three hours before telling police officers that she and Jim had come across two strangers while out boating. It was too dark to identify them. She saw a flash, saw her husband fall, and then panicking, rowed away. She had not told the truth before because she knew her lover would be suspected.

Dr. Dreher was questioned. When informed of Ada's statement, he too admitted being at the scene of the crime, but claimed that Jim Beadle had committed the murder out of loyalty to him. The third member of the unholy trio, Jim Beadle, also admitted being at the scene, but claimed Dr. Dreher had orchestrated the killing and had fired the fatal shots.

All three suspects were arrested and stood trial for the murder of Jim Le Boeuf on July 25, 1927. The murder, because of its eerie setting and the fact that most of the evidence against the accused had come from their own mouths, became a national sensation. The defence offered little in the way of rebuttal.

All three were found guilty. Jim Beadle was sentenced to life imprisonment. Dr. Thomas Dreher, the best-liked man in Morgan City, and Ada Le Boeuf paid for their crime on the gallows.

DR. FRANK LOOMIS
1927

Everyone who ever met Grace Loomis liked her very much. Yet I know for a fact that there was an exception. That person hit Grace flush in the face three times with a blunt instrument, killing her instantly.

We know the exact time the fatal blows were struck. At precisely 9:06 on the night of February 22, 1927, a Detroit telephone operator, diligent Doris McClure, plugged in a telephone line and heard a woman's blood-curdling, terror filled scream. Abruptly the scream stopped. The operator then heard a terse male voice say, "Never mind." The line went dead. Diligent Doris didn't call police, but made a note of the time — 9:06.

At 9:06 p.m. Tom Blockson and Ethel Bell were walking in the street close to Frank and Grace Loomis' home. They heard a loud shriek coming from the house, followed by a windowpane shattering. They thought Dr. Loomis was treating a patient and didn't call police. Tom and Ethel never did explain what type of pain they thought shattered windows.

The cause of all the commotion at the Loomis residence became clear at 9:45. That's when Dr. Frank Loomis ran from his home and summoned his neighbor, Mrs. Mildred Twark, with the unoriginal but nevertheless informative phrase, "My wife has been murdered!"

The doctor and Mildred returned to the Loomis home. Unlike glamorous Hollywood corpses, poor Grace lay in the sun parlor with one leg drawn under her, her neck twisted, and both arms spread out. The upper portion of her body was covered with blood. All in all a horrible sight.

The sun parlor was spattered with blood, reaching to the ceiling. Several pieces of furniture were in odd positions and had obviously been pushed aside during the brief struggle Grace had put up for life.

At Mildred Twark's urging, Dr. Frank checked on his children. Upstairs, Ralph, eight, and Jeanette, five, were fast asleep. The doctor then ran the one block to summon police.

The first officer at the scene asked Dr. Frank, "Did you move anything?", to which the doctor answered, "Yes, and the coroner won't like that. I know this looks bad for me." The officer did a double take.

Senior officials arrived to take Dr. Frank's statement. He told them that he arrived home before 9 o'clock. He talked to his wife briefly, telling her that he was going to take a walk. This was not unusual for the doctor, who was in the habit of taking health walks at every opportunity. Before he left he gave his wife $100 to go shopping for children's clothing the next day.

It was drizzling out. The doctor put on his rubbers and left at exactly 8 o'clock. He outlined his route for detectives and stated that he had arrived back home at 9:45 to find his wife's battered body sprawled in a pool of blood. He had run to her side, put his head to her heart, and at one point attempted to move her to a divan, but gave up. Grace weighed 165 lbs.

It may be noted that the doctor's story accounted for his bloodstained suitcoat, vest and pants. The doctor added his personal theory that maybe a peeping Tom had seen him pass over the $100 to his wife and had killed her six minutes after he left the house. The money was nowhere to be found.

Within 48 hours homicide detectives had pieced together a series of facts which simply didn't jibe with Dr. Frank's theory. For starters, isn't it a bit unusual to take a walk in the rain? Walking slowly, a policeman covered the route taken by the doctor in 34 minutes.

An examination of the Loomis furnace uncovered two pearl shirt buttons. Dr. Frank had been asked to turn over the clothing he had been wearing on the night of the crime. Everything was blood splattered, except for his spotless white shirt. Did the doctor take off his blood-saturated shirt and burn it in the furnace, accounting for the two pearl buttons found there? Police thought so. They also found a fence with two by four stakes attached to fence wire rolled into a coil in the Loomis basement. One of the two by four stakes was missing, which led detectives to believe that the doctor may very well have burned the murder weapon.

Dr. Frank was taken into custody. Investigating officers were sure that the doctor, who was known to have a violent temper, had killed his wife during an argument. If he had not gone for a walk at all, he would have had plenty of time to set up all the physical evidence to fit his story and dispose of the murder weapon in the furnace before dashing over to Mildred Twark's house at 9:45.

Counteracting police theories was the fact that Frank and Grace were a happily married couple. The doctor was a devoted family man with an unblemished reputation. Then there was the little matter of motive. There was absolutely none. Despite police suspicions, Dr. Frank was released from custody.

That isn't to say Frank was home free. Not by a long shot. Detectives followed the doctor in the hope that he would lead them to the motive for killing his wife. Once released, Dr. Frank attended to his most pressing problem first. He buried Grace. After disposing of this pedestrian inconvenience, he led police to one of the oldest motives in the distressing history of murder — the other woman.

Her name was never made public, but we do know juicy tidbits about her. She was not the type of lady one would think would appeal to Dr. Frank. The object of his affection hung around shady bars and loved partying. The doctor visited her every day before his wife's untimely demise. The lady in question would say no more than that she was a good friend and patient of the kindly doctor.

Now equipped with a motive, police arrested Dr. Frank and charged him with his wife's murder. As there was no evidence of premeditation, it was felt that there was no hope of convicting the doctor of first degree murder. At his trial the jury never got to hear that the doctor was having an affair while his wife was alive. No one knows to this day why the unsavory lady wasn't called to testify.

Prosecution attorneys felt that Dr. Frank would crack on the witness stand; the state would accept a manslaughter plea and everyone would be happy. It didn't turn out that way. The doctor was found not guilty.

Dr. Frank was never the same man after his acquittal. He sent his children to their grandparents in Brooklyn, Mich., and concentrated full time on his lady friend. The doctor was completely at his love's mercy. When things went well, which wasn't too often, he was ecstatic. When he had a lovers' quarrel he sank into the depths of depression. His practice suffered until it was nonexistent. He moved frequently. Nothing mattered to him except his girlfriend.

On May 19, 1929, a year after his acquittal, he opened his office at one o'clock in the morning, had a few blasts of whisky, read the Bible, wrote a couple of letters professing his innocence, and hooked himself up to a gas stove. Dr. Frank Loomis was found dead at 8:30 that same morning.

DR. HAROLD GUILFOYLE
1928

Given the right set of circumstances, even the most intimate little dinner parties have been known to deteriorate to bloody murder.

Come along with me now back to 1928. Together we will attend a dinner party thrown by Mrs. Harold Guilfoyle of Hartford, Conn. Mrs. Guilfoyle, together with her doctor husband, Harold, lived in a comfortable upstairs flat at 691 Maple Ave.

The dinner party was being held in honor of Claire Gaudet of New Haven. Claire had arrived in Hartford to attend to legal matters pertaining to her late father's will. That inconsiderate gentleman had died, leaving his estate of over half a million dollars to charity and three old cronies. Claire was attempting to have the will overthrown. She attended the dinner party with her five-year-old daughter, Patricia.

Claire, who was pretty as a picture, if somewhat overweight, had been carrying on a torrid affair with Dr. Guilfoyle for years. Harold was a rascal. There are those who say that he revealed every detail of his dalliances with Claire to his dear wife. Don't go away, our intimate little party warms up appreciably.

Also at the dinner party that night were Algernon Sidney Way, better known as Sid to his friends and his wife. You couldn't miss Sid in a crowd. He had only one arm and a withered side. Sid and Claire also had a little something going between them. Maximin Gaudet, Claire's everloving husband, was back in New Haven. Let's leave him there for now, but he does show up later on.

There you have the guest list — the Guilfoyles, the Ways, Claire Gaudet and little Patricia. Medium rare steaks were served with Idaho baked potatoes. The men puffed on Havanas as they sipped their Courvoisier. All the while both men cast anticipatory glances at the ever willing Claire while the two wives seethed with jealousy.

At 9:30 p.m. it was time for the guests to leave. As they prepared to leave, Sid Way suggested that he treat Patricia to an ice cream cone at the drugstore across the street. Patricia was thrilled at the offer, and away the pair went down the stairs and out the front door. Harold volunteered to give Claire and Patricia a lift to the station, where they were planning on catching the train back to New Haven. Mrs. Guilfoyle, spoilsport that she was, offered to go along as well.

Claire threw on her coat and left the apartment, followed by Harold. Mrs. Guilfoyle went into a bedroom to fetch her coat while Mrs. Way waited for her in the living room.

The loud report of three shots echoed from the downstairs hall. Mrs. Guilfoyle and Mrs. Way dashed out to the top of the stairs and stood dumbfounded as they gazed down at the scene below. Claire Gaudet was now a crumpled heap on the hall floor. Harold was staggering about the hall with blood gushing from a bullet wound in his head. A neighbor, Dr. F.L. Benton, was at the scene in minutes. He examined Claire and pronounced her to be near death.

Claire and Harold were removed to the Guilfoyle apartment. It was found that a bullet had entered Harold's skull just above the left eye and had exited just above the left temple. When able to speak, he could only say that he had had the impression that the attacker had left by the back door. In the dimly lit hall he was unable to distinguish whether the attacker had been a man or woman.

Just after the shooting, Sid Way appeared on the scene. He had left Patricia at the drugstore to eat her ice cream from a dish. The store was out of cones. He was lingering outside the front door waiting for the rest of the guests to come down when the shootings occurred. He told police that no one had come out the front door.

About an hour and a half after the shooting Maximin Gaudet arrived at the Guilfoyles. His story was simply that he had taken the train to Hartford with the intention of meeting his wife at the dinner party. He would then accompany her back to New Haven. As his train was late in arriving, he decided to eat in a restaurant and pick up Claire and Patricia later. Maximin Gaudet didn't seem surprised at his wife's predicament. He told police that considering his wife's lifestyle, it was to be expected.

The investigation continued into the wee hours of the morning. A search was conducted for the murder weapon in the hall and outside the building, but nothing turned up. Finally, the Guilfoyle's apartment was searched with more positive results. A pearl handled .38 calibre revolver was found in a chest of drawers in the living room. Three cartridges had been fired, and eventually this revolver proved to be the attacker's weapon. When questioned Guilfoyle verified that the gun was his. He usually kept it in either his car or in the chest of drawers where it was found. He couldn't say for sure where it was on the night of the shooting. Now it was obvious that the assailant was probably someone who had attended the dinner party that night and had returned the gun to the chest of drawers. At 10:30 the next morning Claire Gaudet died from her wounds.

There you have it. Six people attended a dinner party. One is dead and one is seriously wounded. That leaves four suspects. Let's eliminate five-year-old Patricia, but we had better add Maximin Gaudet. After all, he could have arrived earlier than he said, lurked in the hall and observed Way and Patricia leaving for ice cream. Did he wait for his wife and lover to walk down the steps before shooting them? Did he then make his way out the back door? Gaudet had a motive. He hated his wife and her lover for cheating on him.

Then again, maybe Gaudet was telling the truth. It could have been Way who, after leaving Patricia eating her ice cream, returned to the dimly lit hall, shot Claire and Harold, and then left the premises, only to rush in again a short time later. Did he realize Guilfoyle was winning the competition for Claire's affection and decide to kill them both?

Mrs. Guilfoyle and Mrs. Way? Well, it's difficult to suspect the two ladies. They would have to have been partners in the crime, but then again in the murder business nothing is impossible. They both hated Claire with a passion.

Who killed Claire Gaudet? Don't feel bad if you're having trouble with this one. The Hartford police gave up after five weeks and turned the case over to the county detective Edward J. Hickey.

Hickey decided that since there was a limited number of suspects he would try to locate the killer's position at the time of the murder by the location of the three bullets extracted from the wall. The first bullet struck Claire in the upper back and travelled downward through her body, lodging in the hall wall four feet from the floor. As the bullet was not deflected by bone, Hickey could place the assailant on the stairway behind Claire. The second bullet did not pass through human flesh. From its position in the wall the detective was able to state that this bullet was fired from the same position.

The third bullet was fired from a completely different position. At precisely five-feet, four-inches from the floor, it penetrated the wall horizontally. Guilfoyle was five-feet, eight-inches tall. The bullet was fired four inches lower than the crown of his skull and entered the wall exactly five-feet, four inches from the floor. The wound could have been self-inflicted.

When confronted with this theory, Guilfoyle confessed. Claire was tiring of him and he couldn't bear to lose her. He killed her just as Hickey had described and then turned the gun on himself, intending to commit suicide. In the confusion after the killing he had placed the gun back in the chest of drawers. When he found out everyone but him was suspected of the shooting, he decided to let matters take their own course.

Dr. Harold Guilfoyle was sentenced to life imprisonment in the Connecticut State Prison at Wethersfield. Detective Edward Hickey went on to become commissioner of the Connecticut State Police.

DR. BENJAMIN KNOWLES
1928

Today, the tiny country is known as the Republic of Ghana. Back in 1928, it was a small jewel in the crown of British colonies on the west coast of Africa called Ashanti.

The resident doctor in the town of Bekawi was Dr. Benjamin Knowles. The good doctor and his wife lived in apparent harmony until 4:30 p.m., on October 20, 1928. That was the day someone shot Mrs. Knowles directly in, for want of a better word, the buttocks.

The Knowles' houseboy heard the shot and rushed to the home of Mr. Thortref Margin, the district commissioner. Margin was greeted at the Knowles front door by the doctor, who assured him everything was all right. Margin continued on to take part in a scheduled tennis match.

When he returned from tennis, he learned the houseboy had called on him again, leaving the message, "Missie cry very much."

Next morning, Margin reported the incident to Knowles' superior, Dr. Gush. Knowles told him there had been an accident. He showed Dr. Gush black and blue bruises on his knees and shins where, he claimed, his wife had struck him with an Indian club.

Dr. Gush found Mrs. Knowles standing up in her bedroom. She told him she had been wounded and invited him to examine the wound in her left buttock. The bullet had travelled upward and exited out of the right side of her abdomen.

Mrs. Knowles told Gush that she had been examining her husband's .455 Webley revolver. She placed in on a chair and later sat on the weapon and accidentally discharged it while trying to remove the gun.

Gush had Mrs. Knowles removed to a hospital and three days after the shooting, she died. Her husband was charged with her murder as the police firmly believed she went to her death protecting him.

Two .455 calibre bullets were found in the Knowles cottage. Bullet number one was found by a houseboy on the eve of the shooting in a pool of blood in the bedroom. Bullet number two was found in a wardrobe. There was a scorched hole in mosquito netting draped over the Knowles' bed, and a hole in the wardrobe door.

A search of the home uncovered a loaded .455 Webley revolver with only one discharged cartridge shell. On November 13, 1928, Dr. Knowles' murder trial took place in Kumasi before a lone judge.

The prosecution claimed bullet number two was fired by Dr. Knowles as he lay in bed. They speculated it travelled through the mosquito netting, his wife's body and the wardrobe door, then fell to the base of the wardrobe. They further claimed the doctor attempted to treat his wife's wound, thereby keeping the shooting a secret.

Dr. Knowles stated bullet number two was fired by his wife weeks earlier to frighten him. Bullet number one, the one found in the pool of blood, was the bullet which accidentally killed his wife.

Defence lawyers stated they traced the trajectory of bullet number two. In order for Mrs. Knowles to have been shot by her husband, she would have to have been standing on a chair or Knowles would have to be lying on the floor, both rather farfetched possibilities.

The prosecution countered by stating the fatal shot could have been fired as Mrs. Knowles bent over. If this was the case, how did that other bullet find its way into the pool of blood on the floor?

The perplexing case was decided by the lone presiding

judge, who found Dr. Knowles guilty and sentenced him to death. Dr. Knowles appealed. His conviction was set aside because the presiding judge had not considered manslaughter as an alternative charge to murder. The good doctor was freed and never tried again.

Dr. Knowles died of natural causes in 1933 and took the riddle of the extra bullet to his grave.

DR. PIERRE BOUGRAT
1929

When it comes to murders based on affairs of the heart, it seems there is no one quite like the French. Frenchmen display a certain style and elan toward their amours which is difficult to duplicate.

Take Dr. Pierre Bougrat as a classic example. At 32, Doc had a terrific practice in Aix, France, a gorgeous wife and a big home. To the casual observer it appeared that the young doctor had the world by the tail, but as you and I know, outward appearances are sometimes deceiving. In the doctor's case his wife left a lot to be desired in the love making department. Truth is she simply did not want to perform frequently enough to suit her husband.

Pierre looked elsewhere for his kicks. He discovered that in Marseilles, only about 30 kilometres from Aix, there was an abundance of houses which were not homes. The doctor found out that he could change out of his respectable clothing into the sloppy garb of the waterfront district, and have a barrel of fun every night.

Things went along famously for about a year, or until the frigid wife, suspecting that all was not kosher, put a private eye on Pierre. The detective reported back to Mrs. B. that her husband had a reputation as a real stud among the brothels of Marseilles. Now it so happened that Mrs. B. had an elderly father who thought the sun rose and set on his son-in-law.

In order to save her father from the disgrace of Pierre's philandering, Mrs. B. struck a bargain with her husband. They would continue to live under the same roof, but in the evening they would have separate bedrooms. Pierre was never happier. That night he whistled while he, shall we say, worked down at the waterfront.

Another year went by. Then Mrs. B.'s father died and she no longer had any reason to stay under the same roof with Pierre. She pulled out bag and baggage, and presumably found another roof under which to stay. The doctor found himself the only occupant of his large home in Aix.

At this time in his career, the doctor met a prostitute named Andrea Audibert. It is not quite clear just what made Andrea different from all the other ladies of the night. Whatever, Andrea said try it, you'll like it; and for once in his life Pierre fell in love. He spent every evening with Andrea, partaking of her many charms. There was just one catch. Andrea was owned by a rough, tough, pimp named Marius. The doctor wanted Andrea to stop sharing her favors with utter strangers. He also found that studding around all night and doctoring all day was just too taxing on his constitution. He wanted to install Andrea as his housekeeper in his home in Aix. He decided to buy his true love's freedom from her pimp. The doctor was a bit shocked at the price of the merchandise. Marius wanted 9,000 francs, and Pierre had no choice; he promised Marius he would raise the money.

As luck would have it, one of the doctor's patients back in Aix was the paymaster of a local steel mill. Macques Rumebe visited the doctor each week for an injection. Over the years Rumebe and the doctor became familiar with each other's routine. It was an easy matter for the doctor to reschedule Rumebe's appointment to a day when the paymaster picked up the payroll from the bank and carried it to the mill. The doctor's office was situated between the bank and the mill. It was quite natural for Rumebe to pick up the payroll and drop into the doctor's office for his injection.

With a jaunty walk and a twinkle in his eye Rumebe entered Dr. Bougrat's office for his injection. He received a shot of arsenobenzol and was deader than a mackerel in a matter of minutes.

Rather unimaginatively, the doctor nailed Rumebe upright in a closet and sealed the door. Later he had some wallpaper hangers come in and paper over the hole thing.

Speedy Pierre scampered down to Marseilles, paid Marius 9,000 francs and returned to Aix with his new housekeeper, Andrea. In the meantime, Rumebe had been missed in a matter of hours. There were two schools of thought. He had either met with foul play, or had absconded with his company's payroll. Dr. Bougrat made sure which way the wind blew. He wrote to Rumebe's employer. In disguised handwriting he informed them that Rumebe had been leading a double life and had been carrying on a love affair with a prostitute in Marseilles.

In the routine investigation which followed, the police called on Dr. Bougrat to question him about his patient, Rumebe. The detective was shown into the house by Andrea. The officer couldn't get the nagging feeling out of his head that he had seen Andrea before. When he returned to the police station he spent several hours going through pictures of girls suspected of a variety of crimes. Sure enough, there she was, the Marseilles prostitute, Andrea Audibert.

With his curiosity now aroused, the detective started to track down the route by which a Marseilles prostitute became a doctor's housekeeper in Aix. It wasn't difficult to uncover that the doctor had paid the pimp Marius 9,000 francs on the day Rumebe disappeared. Had the doctor killed the paymaster in order to obtain the money to purchase Andrea's freedom? The detective was sure he was on the right track. Where could the doctor have disposed of the body so quickly before Rumebe was missed? The officer deduced that the body must be somewhere on the doctor's premises. He only had to find evidence of recent renovations and he was sure he would find the body. On his next visit to the doctor's house he was proved correct in every detail.

Dr. Bougrat was arrested and tried for murder. The cagey doctor admitted everything except murder. He claimed he had inadvertently given an overdose to his patient and that the entire affair had been a horrible accident. After he discovered his mistake he had panicked and nailed poor Rumebe up in the closet.

The intriguing story saved Pierre's neck from falling victim to Dr. Guillotine's diabolical machine. He was sentenced to life imprisonment on Devil's Island.

Pierre was sent to the infamous prison in 1929. He was soon recognized by both inmates and officials of the famous penal colony as an extremely capable physician. He became a trustee, and after serving almost six years, he was allowed a month's freedom in the town of St. Laurent du Maroni on the French Guinea mainland. Although he was still under a loose guard the situation was not escape proof.

The first thing Pierre did was to find a woman, and after six years who can blame him. Her name was Annette du Bois, and she turned out to be a real peach. After teaming up with Annette the doctor made up his mind never to return to Devil's Island. To make matters even better Annette had some loot of her own stashed away and she was willing to go anywhere with Pierre.

Annette and Pierre slipped aboard a Dutch freighter heading for Venezuela. The cagey medic had noted that Venezuela didn't have an extradition treaty with France. Sly fox that he was, he pulled it off. Once in Venezuela he found out that he could get a licence to practise medicine in Caracas.

Believe it or not, Pierre married Annette, and set up housekeeping in Caracas. In time he built up a lucrative medical practice and became a respected doctor once again. For nine years Dr. Bougrat practised medicine by day and faithfully returned to his wife's side by night.

In 1944 Dr. Bougrat, a man who had crammed a lot of living into his 53 years, died of a fever epidemic which he was helping to fight.

DR. JAMES SNOOK
1929

Alice and Beatrice Bustin, two Ohio State University students, had reason to be concerned. Their roommate, Theora K. Hix, had left their room at the women's residence on campus at about 7 p.m. on a warm June evening in 1929. She never returned. Next day, with no word from Theora, the two sisters reported her absence to police.

When detectives read the missing persons report, they knew there was no need to search further for Theora Hix. Earlier that day her body had been found in deep grass behind a shooting range about five miles northwest of Columbus, Ohio.

The 24-year-old second year premedical student had been stabbed many times. She had also received several blows about the head, possibly inflicted by a ballpeen hammer. Her jugular vein and her carotid artery had been slashed. Strangely enough, three fingers on her right hand were crushed. The victim had not been sexually attacked.

Alice and Beatrice Bustin were questioned extensively, but could shed little light on their roommate's private life. Theora was a quiet girl who kept to herself. As far as they knew she had no boyfriends. However, they told detectives she had the habit of leaving their room each evening at about 5 p.m. and not returning until after 10 p.m. Knowing that Theora was a very private person, the Bustin sisters never inquired about her absences and Theora never volunteered any information.

An examination of the victim's body indicated that she had met her death sometime before a heavy rain had fallen on Thursday, the night before her body was found. The time of death was further narrowed by Constable John Guy, who was at the shooting range that Thursday evening.

Guy stated that up until 8 p.m. the shooting range was being used by two competing shooting teams. From 8 p.m. to 10 p.m. the range was deserted. At 10 p.m. Guy had concealed himself in an adjoining field in order to apprehend thieves who were stealing livestock from a nearby farm. Had the murder taken place after 10 p.m., Guy would have witnessed it.

Around 10:20 p.m., there was a heavy rain shower. Guy discontinued his surveillance. Since the victim had been killed before the rainfall, it was reasonable to assume that the murder had taken place between 8 and 10 p.m. on Thursday night.

Unknown to Theora's friends, she was keeping company with a man. This fact was revealed to authorities when a university instructor, after being promised anonymity, came forward with the information that he had often seen her driving with Dr. James Howard Snook in the doctor's blue Ford.

Dr. Snook was an unlikely suspect. The lean, balding, bespectacled 50-year-old Snook was a professor of veterinary medicine on the medical facility at Ohio State University. He was married and had an exemplary reputation.

Snook had an interesting hobby. He was an excellent pistol shot, having represented the U.S. at the 1920 Olympics. At one time he was a world champion, and on six occasions was U.S. champion.

When questioned, Snook remained aloof from his interrogators, answering all questions in a curt, brief manner. He immediately admitted having known Theora Hix for three years and volunteered that for some time he had assisted her in paying her university tuition. They often went for drives together in his car and she was an intelligent, interesting conversationalist. Dr. Snook assured detectives that there was nothing further to their relationship.

Columbus police were positive they had their man, but the good doctor was admitting nothing. Then the unexpected happened. Mrs. Smalley, an astute lady who rented furnished rooms on Hubbard Ave., saw photographs of Dr. Snook and Theora Hix in the local newspaper. She had quite a story to tell.

Four months earlier, on February 11, 1929, Dr. Snook had rented a room from Mrs. Smalley, supposedly for himself and his wife. The doctor arranged with Mrs. Smalley that his wife would do the day to day cleaning of the room, while she would give the place a good cleaning once a week. In the four months Dr. Snook and Theora occupied the room, Mrs. Smalley caught a glimpse of Theora only once. She remembered her as she was impressed by the age difference between the doctor and his wife.

Mrs. Smalley went on to state that on the Friday Theora's body was found behind the firing range, Dr. Snook told her he had to leave the city immediately. His wife would be staying until Sunday to wind up their affairs. While Mrs. Smalley wished Dr. Snook good luck, Theora Hix's unidentified body lay in a Columbus funeral home.

Dr. Snook proved to be one cool cucumber. The first hint that his iron-like composure wasn't emotion free occurred when Mrs. Smalley was brought into his presence. Without hesitation she said, "Good evening, Mr. Snook." Snook replied, "Good evening, Mrs. Smalley."

It was story changing time. Dr. Snook admitted that he had set up the little love nest with Theora, but vehemently denied any involvement in her death.

Now hot on the trail, Columbus detectives discovered

that Snook had taken a suit to a dry cleaning establishment on the day Theora's body was found. The suit was examined. There were bloodstains on the jacket sleeves and the knees of the trousers. The blood type was the same as Theora's.

While Mrs. Snook looked on helplessly, police raked through ashes taken from her furnace. They recovered bits of fabric, which they were able to prove came from pyjamas owned by the slain girl.

Snook weakened when faced with this overwhelming array of evidence and admitted killing his lover. It was a brief and skimpy confession, hinting that Theora had been a cocaine addict who had badgered him for money on a daily basis. However, an analysis of Theora's internal organs revealed no signs of her having been an addict.

On July 24, 1929, Dr. Snook stood trial for the murder of Theora Hix. Defence attorneys attempted to prove that his confessions had been obtained under duress and that the doctor was insane anyway. No one was buying.

Dr. Snook took the witness stand in his own defence. He told the court that he had attempted to break off his affair with Theora and return to his wife. He said Theora became incensed, cursing and striking him as he drove his car. He stopped, tried to calm her, but then in a rage rained blows to her head with a hammer. Again, no one was buying the doctor's story. The girl had been attacked with knife and hammer. Her jugular had been severed by the deliberate stroke of a knife. Dr. Snook did clear up one minor mystery. Theora had incurred the three crushed fingers when he accidentally slammed the car door on her hand.

Dr. James Howard Snook was found guilty of murder. On February 28, 1930, he was executed in the electric chair, courtesy of the State of Ohio.

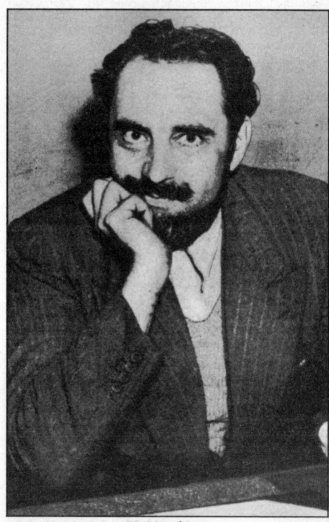

Dr. Marcel Petiot

DR. MARCEL PETIOT
1930

Rarely has a more despicable character taken his place on the stage of criminal infamy than Dr. Marcel Petiot.

Petiot was born in the picturesque French town of Auxerre. He grew up to be a bright, handsome young man. In 1921 he obtained his medical degree and by 1924 had acquired a general practice in Villeneuve. His practice soon became the most prosperous in town. Dr. Petiot was so popular in the community that he was elected mayor in 1925. That same year, he married Georgette Lablais, the daughter of a wealthy Paris restaurant owner. A year later, their son Gerard was born.

In the years which followed Petiot had several brushes with the law. Once he was convicted of fixing an electrical meter, enabling him to obtain free light and power. He was found guilty of this charge, received a suspended sentence and was forced to resign as mayor. On another occasion, he was accused of stealing gasoline from a garage. The charge wasn't pressed.

In 1930, the good doctor was accused of a far more serious crime. A Mme. Debeuve was found strangled to death in a dairy she operated. The place had been robbed. Dr. Petiot had been seen near the dairy at the time of the crime and was strongly suspected of Mme. Debeuve's murder. He was never charged, but from the time of the murder rumors of his involvement spread throughout the town. By 1933 the rumors had become so intense that Petiot moved to Paris and opened a general practice at 66 Rue Caumartin.

Seven years after his arrival in Paris, Petiot purchased a

15-room villa in the Rue Le Sueur near the Arc de Triomphe. He supervised extensive alterations to the villa, including an oversize furnace and a high wall around the garden. To the curious, the doctor explained that he had opened a mental institution at Rue Le Sueur while retaining his home and general practice at Rue Caumartin.

One of Petiot's first patients at his new address was Denise Hotin. Denise had heard that the doctor would perform abortions. After her abortion, she returned to her home village, but for reasons of her own went back to Paris to see Dr. Petiot. No one saw Denise after that. A few inquiries were made from her village, but nothing of an official nature was done. Germany had invaded France and occupied Paris. It was wartime; anything could have happened.

Dr. Petiot let it be known that he would supply drugs to addicts from his new office. His illicit drug trade kept a steady stream of cash pouring in. One fine day, a pimp named van Bever caused a fuss when the doctor refused to sell him dope on credit. Van Bever threatened to tell police of the doctor's drug business. A short while later, van Bever simply disappeared off the face of the earth. His friends figured he had fallen into the hands of the German secret police.

In 1942, Dr. Petiot hatched a diabolical plot which was to place him in a category as one of the most despicable multiple murderers in a world that has far too many vile killers. Realizing that those of the Jewish faith were fleeing France in the face of increasing persecution at the hands of the Germans, the wily Dr. Petiot posed as a man who had the connections to pay off authorities and pave the way out of the country for those in danger.

His first customer was a neighbor, Joachim Gruschinov. In the strictest confidence, Dr. Petiot told his neighbor that he was a member of the Resistance and could get him out of the country for a price. He assured

Gruschinov that not a penny went to the Resistance or to himself. The complete amount was used to pay off officials. Gruschinov gathered together all his valuables and delivered them to Dr. Petiot, who assured him they would be sent to South America in advance of his arrival.

Gruschinov kissed his wife goodbye and promised to send for her as soon as possible. He entered Dr. Petiot's surgery, never to be seen again. Next day, Dr. Petiot told Gruschinov's wife that her husband was on his way to South America.

Dr. Paul Braunberger paid one million francs for his safe passage out of the country. He too told his wife he would be sending for her after he settled in Spain. Dr. Braunberger was never heard of again.

M. and Mme. Kneller and their eight-year-old son walked into Dr. Petiot's surgery and disappeared off the face of the earth.

In 1943, Petiot had a narrow escape. Pierre Beretta, an escaped prisoner of war, had made arrangements to flee France with Petiot's help. When he was picked up by the Gestapo, he squealed on Petiot to save his own skin.

Dr. Petiot was taken into custody by the Gestapo. Scared sick, he decided to play his one trump card. He confessed to murder, but pointed out that all his victims had been Jewish. The Gestapo checked out the identities of his victims and, after detaining him for six months, set him free. Dr. Petiot had correctly read his adversaries. The Germans felt the sleazy doctor was doing their dirty work for them.

Dr. Petiot returned to his wife and his practice. Numerous men, women and children fell into his net. He made millions of francs during his two-year killing spree. Initially, Petiot dissolved bodies in lime, but when this material became difficult to procure, he dissected them and burned them in his large furnace. It wasn't that difficult. His unsuspecting victims placed themselves totally in his care. They trustingly accepted the anti-typhoid injection he gave them, never for an instant realizing that it was a deadly poison.

On March 11, 1944, Dr. Petiot's chimney caught fire. A neighbor, Mme. Marcais, observed flames shooting out of the chimney. The odor of the smoke was nauseating. She called police, who in turn called the fire department. Firemen broke into the large rambling villa and made their way into the furnace room. They stopped short. There on the floor around the furnace were the arms, legs, torsos and heads of Petiot's victims.

Police searched an adjoining garage, where they uncovered a vast array of clothing and personal effects. They also found Petiot's death book, complete with names and addresses. The death list was headed with the word "Escapes."

French detectives descended on Petiot's home on Rue Caumartin, but the bird had flown. He had deposited his wife and child in his home town of Auxerre and had returned to Paris, where he hid out in a friend's house. The gruesome discovery of the doctor's victims was front page news until June 6, when the Allied landing in Normandy took over the news. On August 24, Paris was liberated and Petiot and his horrible crimes were again reported by the country's press.

Word was received by the police that Petiot might have joined the Resistance using a false name. A sample of his handwriting was checked against the handwriting of members of the Resistance who had joined since June 6. It was a long shot, but it paid off. Petiot's handwriting was identified as that of a Capt. Witterwald. On November 2, 1944, the Resistance turned over the bogus captain to the police.

On March 18, 1946, Dr. Petiot stood trial for the murders of 27 individuals killed at Rue Le Sueur. Petiot swore he had been working on behalf of the Resistance and that all his victims had been German soldiers and collaborators. His story didn't wash with the French jury. The sensational trial lasted 16 days, but the jury took only two hours to find Petiot guilty of 24 counts of murder.

In an attempt to save their client's life, defence attorneys appealed to the president of France for clemency. Their plea was rejected. On May 26, 1946, Dr. Marcel Petiot was put to death with the assistance of a contraption invented by another French doctor named Guillotine.

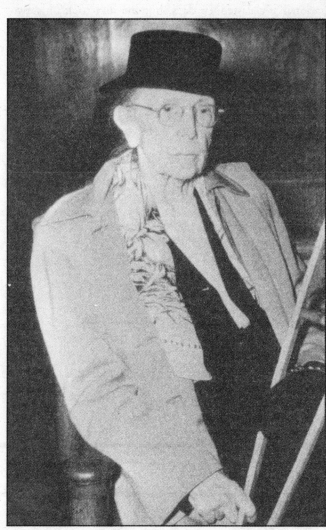

Dr. Alice Wynekoop

DR. ALICE WYNEKOOP
1933

One of the most unusual and, at the same time, interesting individuals ever to stand accused of murder, has to be Dr. Alice Wynekoop. For one thing, Alice was old enough to know better. She was 63 in 1933 when she pulled the trigger.

Frank and Alice Wynekoop were medical doctors, who lived in a large, rambling custom-built home at 3406 W. Monroe St. in Chicago. During their happy years, the Wynekoops had three children. Walter, the eldest Wynekoop, became a successful businessman. He married, moved to the suburbs, and doesn't enter our story. The second child, Earle, was his mother's favorite from birth. Earle was no good. We'll get back to him later. Catherine, the youngest child, following in her parents' footsteps, became a respected medical doctor.

Unfortunately, Frank Wynekoop died before his children reached adulthood. It fell to his wife Alice to raise the children. She was quite a lady. Alice continued to practise medicine from her well-equipped office in the basement of her spacious home. Not only did she raise her children, she also found time away from her busy practice to work diligently for several charities.

While Catherine and Walter grew up to be honest, hard-working individuals who eventually moved out of the Monroe St. home, Earle was quite another kettle of fish. Earle was in his early twenties when he married 18-year-old Rheta Gardner of Indianapolis. Because Earle was unable to support himself, let alone a wife, Alice converted the third floor of her home into an apartment for the young couple. The mansion on Monroe had one other occupant, Enid Hennessey, a middle-aged schoolteacher who had roomed at the Wynekoops with her elderly father. When her father died, Enid stayed on.

Rheta was not happy. She had several fair to middling reasons. First of all, what young bride wants to live under the same roof with her mother-in-law? Then there was Earle's habit of spending a lot of time away from home. It was an open secret that he habitually played the field with other ladies. On top of all this, Rheta was a bit of a hypochondriac, forever complaining of a variety of aches and pains.

Things came to a head on the evening of November 21, 1933. At about 10 p.m., police were called to the Wynekoop home. Enid Hennessey and Alice met them at the door. Dr. Alice said, "Something terrible has happened; come on downstairs and I will show you."

Once downstairs, police were faced with the eerie sight of beautiful young Rheta Wynekoop lying on an operating table. Her nude body was wrapped in a thick blanket. The dead girl's clothing lay in a bundle beside the table. When the blanket was removed, a bullet hole was discovered in the girl's breast. Under a cloth on the operating table, police found a .32 calibre Smith and Wesson revolver. The girl's face appeared to be slightly burned.

Dr. Wynekoop said something about money and drugs being missing from the house. She thought robbers might be responsible. No one took the doctor's theory very seriously.

Naturally enough, police were anxious to chat with the deceased woman's husband. Earle was pursuing his latest attempt at making a living. He was on a train headed for the Grand Canyon, supposedly to take photographs. Notified of his wife's untimely demise, the grieving husband returned, a shapely brunette draped over his arm. When asked the identity of the lady, Earle told reporters that his little address book held the names of 50 more just like her. Earle suggested that some moron must have killed Rheta. He admitted that his marriage was a failure and volunteered that his wife was mentally ill. Earle didn't impress anyone.

When it became obvious that Earle the cad could not have killed his wife, police directed their attention to the victim's frail mother-in-law, Alice Wynekoop. Under intensive questioning, Dr. Alice confessed. She stated that Rheta had always been concerned about her health. She disrobed each day to weigh herself. Early on the afternoon of her death, the doctor had walked in on Rheta, who was sitting nude on the operating table. She had just weighed herself and was complaining of a severe pain in her side.

Dr. Wynekoop suggested that since Rheta had already disrobed, it was a convenient time for her to be examined. The doctor thought that a few drops of chloroform might ease the discomfort. Rheta breathed deeply from a chloroform-soaked sponge. Dr. Wynekoop inquired if her patient was still experiencing discomfort. She received no reply. Rheta wasn't breathing. Dr. Wynekoop tried artificial respiration without success. Rheta was dead.

Alice Wynekoop claimed that she panicked. It was a known fact that Rheta and Earle were not getting along, and that there was a great deal of ill-feeling between Alice and her daughter-in-law. Who would believe the freak death? There was a loaded revolver in the room. Holding it about six inches from the nude body, the doctor fired into the lifeless corpse.

Chicago detectives simply didn't believe Dr. Wynekoop's story. The doctor was arrested and charged with murder. Due to the accused's poor health, the trial was delayed several times. When it finally took place, things didn't go at all well for the good doctor.

From the witness stand, Enid Hennessey related details

of the events of that fateful day. She had returned to the Wynekoop home about six that evening. Alice put pork chops on the stove for dinner. The two friends discussed literature. There was a place setting at the table for Rheta. Alice explained that Rheta had gone downtown at about three that afternoon and had not returned. That seemed strange to Enid. Rheta's coat and hat were hanging in full view.

After dinner, Enid and Alice chatted in the library. When Enid complained of hyperacidity, Alice volunteered to go down to her office to fetch some pills. It was then that the doctor discovered the body of her daughter-in-law.

Hold the phone! Something's wrong. According to Alice's own confession, Rheta was dead early in the afternoon. Did Alice calmly await her friend's return, cook up pork chops, chat about books, knowing all the while that Rheta lay dead in the basement? For shame!

The prosecution had a few other damaging tidbits. A post mortem indicated that Rheta had died as a result of the bullet wound. The body was exhumed. The burning about the face was caused by powder burns, not chloroform. In fact, Rheta's body held no traces of chloroform.

The prosecution proved through the evidence of several witnesses that Dr. Alice always thought that Earle had entered a poor marriage. Rheta was not good enough for her boy. To add frosting to the cake, she had recently insured Rheta's life.

An Illinois jury deliberated 14 hours before bringing in a guilty verdict. Dr. Wynekoop was sentenced to life imprisonment and was incarcerated in the Women's Reformatory at Dwight, Ill. After serving over 15 years, she was paroled in 1949 at age 78. Dr. Alice Wynekoop died two years after her release from prison.

DR. BUCK RUXTON
1936

Susan Johnson did what many people do when they stroll over a country bridge. She absently looked down at the meandering stream below. Could that be a human arm protruding from some newspapers on the river bank? Susan, who was vacationing in Moffat, Scotland, hurriedly returned to her hotel room where she told her brother of her suspicions. He travelled the two miles to the bridge and confirmed his sister's gruesome find. Then he called the police.

What confronted the authorities on that pleasant September afternoon in 1935 was not a pretty sight. The newspapers held the dismembered portions of not one, but two, bodies. There were four individual bundles containing small segments of both bodies. The victims were adult females.

Within the next two days additional parts of the same two bodies were found in the general area of the original four bundles. Complete sections of the two bodies had been cut away in an obvious attempt to hinder identification.

To add an element of mystery to the already strange discovery of two separate dismembered and mutilated bodies, police found a Cyclops eye in one of the newspaper bundles. This phenomenon, known as Cyclopia, is the fusing together of two eyes, which appear as a single eye in the middle of the forehead. This malformation is extremely rare in humans, but does occur more frequently in pigs. In the case of humans, it is usually accompanied by other deformities which result in death a few hours after birth. The name, of course, is derived from a mythical race of one-eyed giants whose chief occupation in Greek mythology was the manufacture of thunderbolts for Zeus. The human Cyclops eye was a strange and puzzling oddity to discover along a peaceful meandering river in Scotland.

A heavy rainfall had taken place on September 19. It was ascertained that the bodies would have been washed away had they been deposited on the river bank before this date. Police began their investigation by checking out all women reported missing since September 19.

In this routine manner, investigating officers found out that Mary Jane Rogerson, a nursemaid in the home of Dr. Buck Ruxton, had been reported missing weeks before Miss Johnson's gruesome discovery under the bridge. Police were also given to understand that Dr. Ruxton's wife had left him at approximately the same time. Mary Rogerson's mother identified several pieces of clothing found with the bodies as belonging to her daughter. She had sewn a patch into one of the garments herself.

Detectives were already well acquainted with Dr. Buck Ruxton. He had called on them several times in the previous three weeks to complain that his wife had left him, and that he wanted her found and returned. After the gruesome discovery he continued to call on the police, claiming that rumors were being spread connecting him with the bodies found under the bridge. Dr. Ruxton stated that the rumors were ruining his practice and must be stopped.

Police were not ready to act. Mrs. Ruxton had not been identified as a victim and, while Dr. Ruxton was strongly suspected of complicity in the murder, police found it prudent to wait until positive identification could be established. I must point out that visual examination of the bodies was ruled out as a method of identification. The mutilations to both bodies were so extensive that it was impossible to identify the bodies in this way.

Dr. Ruxton was born in Bombay, India. Thankfully he had his name changed from Bukhtyar Rustomji Ratanji Hakim to Buck Ruxton. He received his medical degree from the University of Bombay, and later specialized in surgery at the same university. He had maintained a comfortable home at 2 Dalton Square, Lancaster, since 1930, where he carried on a rather successful medical practice.

Mrs. Ruxton was the former Isabella Kerr. She had been married once before in 1919. After meeting Dr. Ruxton, she had her marriage dissolved, and married the doctor in 1928.

During the seven years of their marriage, Mrs. Ruxton and the doctor argued and fought incessantly. Dr. Ruxton was insanely jealous, and often unjustly accused her of having affairs with other men. Ruxton had a short temper and often struck his wife.

His diary reveals that they always kissed and made up. Theirs was an unhappy household.

The Ruxtons had three children, aged six, four, and two. Mary Rogerson, their nursemaid, was 20. Mary rarely left the Ruxton residence during the week. Usually she spent her day off with her parents. She had never been late for an appointment, nor had she ever stayed out overnight without informing her family. Neither Mrs. Ruxton nor Mary were seen by anyone after September 14, 1935.

Three women, other than Mary, worked at the good doctor's home. Mrs. Agnes Oxley, a charwoman, worked at 2 Dalton Square every day of the week, except Saturday, starting at 7:10 a.m. Mrs. Elizabeth Curwen also showed up every day starting at 8:30 a.m. and staying until her work was completed. A third woman, Mrs. Mabel Smith, had only recently been hired on a part-time basis, working Monday through Thursday from 2 p.m. to 7 p.m. The work schedules of these women later proved to be of crucial importance.

On Friday, September 13, Mrs. Curwen was told by Dr. Ruxton not to return until the following Monday. On Sunday, the 15th, Mrs. Oxley was surprised to find Dr. Ruxton at her doorstep at 6:30 a.m., advising her not to come to work. He told her that Mrs. Ruxton and Mary had gone on a holiday to Edinburgh. Mrs. Smith was not due at Dalton Square until Monday.

Dr. Ruxton had managed to dismiss his three employees, leaving him alone in his home on Friday night, Saturday and Sunday.

All that weekend Ruxton scurried about. To everyone who met him he appeared agitated and nervous. As his car was in for repairs, he hired a vehicle and placed his children with friends.

When the charwomen reported for work the following week they found two upstairs bedrooms locked. The house had undergone many changes over the weekend. The walls along the stairway appeared to be blood splattered. Rugs had been taken up and thrown into the backyard. These, too, had large brown stains. The doctor magnanimously gave the rugs to Mrs. Oxley and Mrs. Curwen. He explained that he had severely cut his hand while opening a tin of fruit, accounting for the bloodstains on the wall and rug. He also told them that he was preparing the house to be redecorated. The ladies worked hard all that week cleaning up.

To everyone, even those who didn't inquire, Dr. Ruxton gave conflicting stories about his wife's and Mary's sudden departure. To some he stated that Mary was pregnant, and that his wife had gone away with her to attempt to terminate the pregnancy. He told others that the two women were on vacation. All week the charwomen cleaned and threw out rubbish. One of them later remembered a bloody piece of cotton wool which the doctor had her burn in the backyard, together with a bloody dress.

On September 19, at 7:30 a.m., Ruxton brought his car around to the back door of his home. As Mrs. Oxley worked out of sight in the kitchen, he made several trips upstairs and back down to his car. After he left, Mrs. Oxley, who was now joined by Mrs. Curwen, noticed that the two upstairs rooms, which had been locked for five days, were now open. The two ladies entered the rooms and remarked on the vile smell emanating from them.

Next day Dr. Ruxton mentioned the smell to the two women. He suggested they buy a bottle of eau de cologne. Mrs. Curwen bought the cologne and gave it to the doctor. Later on the fragrance was much in evidence in the odoriferous rooms.

It must be noted that in the two weeks between September 14 and the discovery of the bodies on September 29, Dr. Ruxton was a busy little boy. He was scurrying around the countryside, trying to establish an alibi, ministering to his patients, placing his children, trying desperately to have his house decorated, and keeping three inquisitive women from finding out the truth while making up stories to account for the absence of his wife and nursemaid. All the while he was dissecting two bodies and disposing of the pieces. It was all enough to tire a man. No wonder everyone who saw him during this period remembers his desperate appearance.

After the bodies were discovered near Moffat, Dr. Ruxton became frantic. He contacted everyone he had seen in the previous two weeks asking them to support him in the story he would be telling the police.

Dr. Buck Ruxton was arrested and charged with the murder of Mary Rogerson on October 15, 1935. Two months later he stood trial for murder at the Manchester Assizes.

Once the arrest was made, police swooped down on 2 Dalton Square and almost took the house apart.

Floorboards and parts of the wall were removed to the Department of Forensic Medicine at Glasgow University. Stains appearing on both wall and floor were identified as human blood. Dr. Ruxton's hand was examined. It was established that a fruit tin could not have inflicted such a wound. The severe cut was self-inflicted by a sharp knife. A local newspaper to which the doctor subscribed was found wrapped around a portion of Mary Rogerson's body. Also found with the body was a section of a sheet, which matched perfectly with the other section found in the doctor's house.

Although the doctor maintained his innocence, it is believed that during one of his frequent fits of temper he killed his wife. Mary Rogerson, the nursemaid, may have witnessed the crime and had to be silenced.

Dr. Ruxton was found guilty and sentenced to death. He was hanged at Strangeways Prison on May 12, 1936.

But what of the mysterious Cyclops eye found with the two bodies? Despite many far out theories put forward at Ruxton's trial, it is a mystery which hasn't been solved to this day.

DR. MERRILL JOSS
1941

Doctors Merrill and Laverne Joss were the most respected young couple in the town of Richmond, Maine. Not that much ever happened in Richmond, but all that changed on the evening of March 27, 1941.

That was the night the town's chief of police was called to Dr. Merrill Joss' impressive old colonial home. Dr. Joss met the chief at the door. To say he was distraught would be to understate the case.

"It's my wife," the doctor explained. "She's been attacked by a dope addict or at least that appears to be the case. A bearded stranger appeared at my door demanding narcotics. Naturally, I turned him away. A doctor's house is an easy target, you know."

When the chief asked for a description, the doctor quickly replied, "The man was about five-feet-eight, had shaggy unkempt hair, wore a beard and had a dark coat and cap."

The doctor went on to hurriedly explain that he had left the house to complete an errand and was as far as the railroad tracks when he heard his dog Trixie barking. He returned to the house to find his office burglarized. Alarmed for his wife's safety, he searched the house for her. When he noticed that the door leading off the kitchen into the cellar was open, he dashed downstairs to find his wife lying on the cellar floor, bludgeoned about the head.

All of this was blurted out to the chief as they made their way through the house and down the cellar stairs. The chief noted blood on the stairs, wall and the floor.

There was Laverne Joss, unconscious. In minutes, Dr. Edwin Pratt joined Dr. Joss, peering over Laverne's still form. Dr. Pratt dressed the head wounds as best he could with some gauze. Joss said that he would drive his wife to the hospital. Pratt insisted that an ambulance be called immediately. There was a tense moment, but Pratt prevailed.

An ambulance sped away to hospital with Laverne, while a horde of detectives and citizens joined in an effort to apprehend the man described by Dr. Joss. In a community the size of Richmond, everyone knew the victim of the wild attack. Both she and her husband were beloved by their friends and neighbors. Both were on a first-name basis with many of the police officers now investigating the burglary and the assault on Laverne. That same night, Dr. Laverne Joss died of her wounds.

Dr. Merrill repeated his story to detectives in detail. Probably it was State Police Lieutenant Leon Shepard who first privately doubted his story. The seasoned detective had never heard of a dope addict knocking at a door and asking for drugs. Buying dope, stealing dope, yes; but walking up to a doctor's residence and simply asking for dope just didn't sit well.

As the extensive search for the shaggy stranger continued, detectives were provided with another piece of information concerning Merrill Joss. Evidently, when Laverne was brought into hospital, a blood transfusion was immediately ordered. Merrill objected, insisting upon a blood cross-matching. Laverne died before any transfusion was attempted. It was noted she had 27 head wounds and that her wedding ring was missing.

When Merrill was questioned about the ring, he confirmed that his wife always wore it and he had no idea how it had disappeared. Astute Lt. Shepard had his own theory. He got down on his hands and knees on the Joss' kitchen floor and, in true *Columbo* fashion, searched for the ring. Sure enough there, underneath the refrigerator, was Laverne's ring.

Now, hot to trot, Shepard examined the cellar. In nearly empty bins of vegetables, he found a watch belonging to Laverne. The wily detective reconstructed the crime in his mind.

Shepard dismissed Merrill's story as a fabrication to cover his own tracks. He theorized that Merrill and Laverne had not been getting along — possibly there was another woman. The pair had argued in the kitchen. Laverne had taken off her ring and had thrown it at her husband. The ring had lodged under the refrigerator.

Merrill had picked up something and struck out at his wife. She had slumped to the floor, unconscious. He then threw her down the cellar steps. As she tumbled down, her wrist hit the wall, flinging the watch into a bin of carrots. Merrill cleaned the blood off the kitchen floor, ransacked his own office and either hid or destroyed the murder weapon before calling police. Shepard's theory accounted for all the known facts, except the 27 wounds on Laverne's head.

Shepard continued his investigation. Laboratory technicians were brought into the house. From the kitchen floor, they extracted tiny cotton threads almost invisible to the naked eye. Elsewhere in the house, they found a cloth which proved to be of the same fibres as those taken from the floor. Someone had wiped the floor clean. Certainly, a dope addict wouldn't have stopped to clean the floor after throwing his victim down the stairs.

Lt. Shepard's suspicions had first been raised by the doctor's implausible story. Now, he checked out the doctor's friends and discovered that Merrill was keeping company with a winsome cook at a local eatery. Elizabeth Mayo was questioned and readily co-operated with police. It was true. She and the doctor were seeing each other on the side, so to speak. Merrill had talked of divorce, but

Elizabeth had never thought he would go as far as killing his wife. She produced love letters written by Merrill only hours before his wife's death. That's called motive, folks.

Detectives made a moulage cast of Laverne's head. They then proceeded to make a cast of the crude cellar floor. They found that by placing the head cast against the cast of the rough floor, they could match the two. Eerily, the wounds on the head cast fit the rough edges of the floor. Laverne had received some of her wounds when she was thrown down the stairs onto the floor.

An examination of the steps uncovered a lone eyebrow hair and minute pieces of flesh. The eyebrow hair matched those taken from Laverne's skull. The impact of her head against the steps may have accounted for several of the head wounds.

The entire case against Merrill was circumstantial, but it added up the way Lt. Shepard figured at the beginning, while boy scouts and police were scouring three counties for a man who didn't exist.

Most of the community were gathered at the Methodist church for 37-year-old Laverne Joss' funeral. Merrill Joss was supported by a galaxy of friends as he dabbed at his eyes with a white handkerchief. As Merrill left the church, he was taken into custody by State Police Chief Henry Weaver. Charged with his wife's murder, he was incarcerated in the Sagadahoc County Jail.

A few weeks later, while awaiting trial, Merrill borrowed a razor blade from another inmate. He cut the skin of his right arm and, using his fingernail, raised an artery. He then cut the artery with the blade. A guard found him unconscious and immediately summoned a physician. He was rushed to hospital and given blood transfusions. Attending physicians managed to save his life.

On June 23, 1941, Dr. Merrill Joss stood trial for his wife's murder. The trial lasted 10 days. Prosecuting attorneys dramatically revealed the history of the Joss' marriage. Both had been married before and had become attracted to each other while working together in a hospital. They had divorced their respective spouses and married each other.

Merrill admitted from the witness stand that he and his wife had not been getting along and had discussed divorce. Although married for over five years, they had never lived as man and wife. Laverne had undergone an operation just before marrying him, which made normal sex impossible. Their married life had been more of a brother/sister relationship than one of husband and wife. He further stated that his wife had been aware of his love for Elizabeth Mayo. Their talk of divorce had been amicable.

Merrill Joss got off relatively easy. The jury evidently felt that the crime did not contain the necessary "malice aforethought" and so reduced their verdict to one of guilty of manslaughter.

On July 5, 1941, Dr. Merrill Joss was sentenced to not less than 10 years and not more than 20 years imprisonment in the State Prison at Thomaston, Maine.

DR. ROBERT CLEMENTS
1947

Dr. Robert George Clements was born in Belfast, Ireland. He became an M.D. in 1904, at age 24. The young general practitioner was a bit different than his colleagues right from the beginning. For one thing the good doctor liked the good life. Clements dined in the best restaurants. He attended the theatre regularly, more often than not with a bright-eyed Irish colleen on his arm. The good life necessitated more funds than the doctor earned at his humble practice, so he was often strapped for ready cash. This situation served to gall the man of medicine, but a sure cure was just around the corner. Her name was Edyth Ann Mercier.

Now Edyth was not your average sweet young thing. She was a good ten years Clements' senior. What's more she was plain. But there were compensating factors. Edyth's daddy was an extremely wealthy grain merchant. On the day of his marriage, Dr. Clements came into a tidy sum of cash. Then, as if on cue, Edyth's daddy died of natural causes 18 months after the marriage. He left Edyth £25,000, a princely sum in 1913.

While there is no proof that Dr. Clements had anything whatsoever to do with his father-in-law's death, you should know, in light of future events, that he was Mr. Mercier's doctor during his last illness. Dr. Clements signed the death certificate, stating cancer to be the cause of death.

The Clements' financial status, now substantially improved, allowed the doctor to partake of the good life he so craved. The couple joined several exclusive social clubs, contributed heavily to reputable charities and, in the main, were considered to be an integral part of Belfast's status-conscious society.

Seven years later, the bloom was definitely off the rose. Edyth was aghast to discover that they, or to be more specific, her husband, had gone through their entire fortune. To add insult to injury, nasty rumors were being bandied about, referring to the doctor's unmedical dalliances with younger lady friends.

Coincidental with their financial and domestic difficulties, Edyth fell ill. Her husband told friends that she suffered from sleeping sickness and that the prognosis was not good. Clements was correct. Edyth died in 1920, leaving the doctor so distraught that he personally signed the death certificate, sold his practice and moved to Manchester.

One thing you can say for Robert George Clements — he was a fast worker. No sooner was his shingle swaying in the Manchester breeze than he was the steady escort of a bevy of that city's most eligible rich ladies. A year after Edyth's death, Clements married for the second time. Mary McCleery, the daughter of a wealthy Manchester industrialist, became wife number two. Once more, the doctor was in the chips. Once more, he spent money with, as they used to say, reckless abandon. Once more, his wife grew ill just as the money was running out. Mary lasted until 1925, when she suddenly expired. Dr. Clements signed the death certificate, listing the cause of death as endocarditis.

Three years later, Dr. Clements went to the well for the third time. Katherine Burke was not of the same mould as numbers one and two. Katherine was not wealthy and was acquainted with Clements' previous wives. There is even a possibility that Clements actually cared for Katherine and there is undeniable evidence that his practice had prospered to the extent that he was able to live in the grand manner without outside help.

155

This state of affairs lasted until 1939. Poor investments in the hotel business reduced Dr. Clements' funds to a dangerously low level. That's when the doctor let it be known that Katherine was suffering from tuberculosis. She died, even after Dr. Clements brought in a young colleague at the last moment. The grieving husband suggested that tuberculosis had carried Katherine away. The young doctor agreed.

For the first time in his murderous career, Dr. Clements was suspected of foul play. A friend of his most recently departed wife was a lady doctor, Dr. Irene Gayus. She personally disliked Clements and when she learned that he had signed the death certificates of his previous two wives, she grew downright ugly. Dr. Gayus ran to the police, suggesting they delay Katherine's burial. However, they were too late. Katherine had been cremated only a few hours before police arrived at the scene.

There is no evidence that Clements had knowledge of this near miss. He went on his merry way. Wife number four was Amy Victoria Barnett, a lady 20 years the doctor's junior. Papa Barnett was loaded. And what's more, he conveniently died in 1940, leaving his daughter and her husband a cool £22,000 and his opulent residence in Southport.

Wouldn't you just know it, seven years later, Dr. Clements was telling his acquaintances that he wife wasn't well at all. He had a colleague, Dr. John Holmes, look in on her, but the doctor couldn't pinpoint the problem. A few evenings later, Dr. Holmes received an urgent call from Dr. Clements that his wife was gravely ill.

Dr. Holmes had the stricken woman admitted to the Astley Bank Nursing Home, where she was immediately examined by Dr. Andrew Brown. Brown noticed that Mrs. Clements' eyes had pinpoint pupils, her skin had turned bluish and she was having difficulty breathing. He thought she was suffering from an overdose of morphine.

Next morning, at 9:30 a.m., Amy Victoria Clements died.

Upon hearing the distressing news, Clements suggested his wife had suffered from a brain tumor. Dr. Brown disagreed and insisted on performing an autopsy immediately. Dr. James Houston, a young pathologist who knew the Clements well, assisted Dr. Brown. The brain was examined, but no evidence of a tumor was found. Dr. Houston, for reasons never explained, destroyed the vital organs he removed from the body. However, he later reported that his testing of blood samples indicated that Mrs. Clements' death was caused by myeloid leukemia.

This conclusion did not sit well with Dr. Brown. He contacted the coroner, who in turn contacted police. The local gendarmes took a long look. When they discovered Dr. Clements had been writing prescriptions for large quantities of morphine for patients who had never been treated with the drug, they decided to act. A second autopsy was ordered, and Dr. Houston was notified of this decision.

When police went to question Dr. Clement, they found him unconscious in his kitchen. He died hours later, leaving behind a short note. The note read: "To Whom it May Concern, I can no longer tolerate the diabolical insults to which I have recently been exposed."

The second post mortem proved to be most revealing. Remember that vital organs had been destroyed, so the pathologist had little to work with. However, he was able to establish that death had been caused by an overdose of morphine. A search of Clements' flat turned up large quantities of morphine tablets hidden in bottles.

A few days later, Dr. Houston was found dead in his laboratory. He had taken 300 times the lethal dose of sodium cyanide. Poor Houston, despondent over wrongly certifying that Mrs. Clements had died of leukemia, had ended it all.

On Tuesday, June 25, 1947, an inquest into the weird events leading successively to the deaths of Mrs. Clements, Dr. Clements and Dr. Houston, was held in Southport. Three days later the jury came to the conclusions that; a) Mrs. Clements was murdered by Dr. Clements; b) Dr. Clements committed suicide; and c) Dr. Houston took his own life in a state of depression. It was learned that Dr. Houston had committed a series of medical errors, which had caused him to become severely depressed. The Clements' case was the last straw.

And so ended the case of the doctor who married and poisoned four wives.

DR. JOHN ADAMS
1950

Dr. John Bodkin Adams, 58, had practised medicine for over 35 years in the resort town of Eastbourne, England. He never married, and lived alone in a large Victorian home with only a housekeeper to care for his needs. The doctor had a lucrative practice and was considered to be a pillar of the community. Yet he was to become the central figure in one of the most sensational murder cases ever to unfold in England.

The doctor's life was to become entwined forever with that of a patient, Mrs. Edith Alice Morell. An elderly lady, Mrs. Morell was visiting her son in Cheshire in June 1948, when she suffered a stroke. Taken to the Cheshire General Hospital, she was in great distress, and was given a quarter grain of morphine each day for the nine days

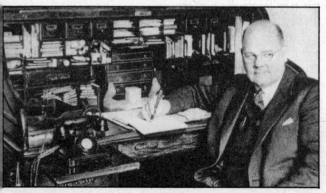

Dr. John Adams

she stayed in hospital. On July 5 she was transferred by ambulance to Eastbourne, where she came under the care of Dr. Adams, who remained her doctor until her death on November 13, 1950, at the age of 81. Mrs. Morell's body was cremated, and that, for all intents and purposes, was that.

Six years passed before any further notice was paid to Mrs. Morell and the manner of her death. In 1956 rumors spread in and around Eastbourne that many of Dr. Adams' patients who had died had left him bequests in their wills. These rumors came to the attention of the authorities and it wasn't long before Scotland Yard dispatched senior investigators to look into Dr. Adams and his medical practice. As a result of their inquiries the doctor was arrested and charged with Mrs. Morell's murder.

The murder case that unfolded captured the imagination of the English-speaking world. While many doctors have stood trial for murder in England, rarely had a doctor been accused of murder while ministering to a patient. In fact, the last such case took place over a hundred years earlier, when the infamous Dr. Palmer of Rugeley was convicted of murder. The Adams trial lasted seventeen days, making it the longest murder trial to take place in England up to that time.

Mrs. Morell's stroke had left her partially paralyzed. Eventually she was able to get around with assistance, but required nurses around the clock. Although the alleged crime was six years old at the time of the trial, the nursing records detailing frequency of injections and quantities of drugs administered were available. All medication, whether injected by the nurses or not, was given under the doctor's instructions.

It was established that Dr. Adams was a beneficiary in Mrs. Morell's will. He stood to gain a prewar Rolls Royce, as well as an amount of silver valued at £275. After Mrs. Morell's death Dr. Adams did, in fact, come into possession of these two items.

From the time Mrs. Morell came under Dr. Adams' care, she received a quarter grain of morphine and a quarter grain of heroin daily. No doubt she became somewhat addicted to the good feeling these drugs gave her, for generally speaking, Mrs. Morell was an irritable and demanding patient.

During September 1950, when Mrs. Morell had only seven weeks to live, her medication was drastically altered by Dr. Adams. He instructed that she be given increased quantities of both morphine and heroin. Mrs. Morell received 10 grains of heroin on November 8, 12 grains on November 9, and 18 on November 11. On November 12, the day before she died, Mrs. Morell received three and a half grains of heroin and two grains of morphine.

Was Mrs. Morell's dosage of these drugs increased in order to end her life or was the doctor doing everything possible to alleviate pain for a dying patient? The line is a thin one, which many physicians have to walk. Maybe it was even thinner in 1950 than it is today.

Other pertinent events that occurred during Mrs. Morell's illness came to light. Dr. Adams had known he was in his patient's will. At one point he had gone to Scotland for a vacation and Mrs. Morell, in a fit of anger, changed her will, leaving him nothing. Later Dr. Adams returned to her good graces and was placed back in her will. There is little doubt that Dr. Adams was concerned about his patient's will. He had discussed the matter with Mrs. Morell's lawyer on several occasions, and at one point suggested that the lawyer draw up a new will and get Mrs. Morell's son to agree to it at a later date. Mrs. Morell's lawyer turned down such a shady proposition.

Conversely, there was the matter of the competent nurses who took care of Mrs. Morell during her long illness. Not one of them spoke up or suggested that during her last weeks Mrs. Morell's dosage was too high. Even

Dr. Adams' partner, Dr. Harris, who filled in for his colleague while he was in Scotland, continued the regime of morphine and heroin. His explanation was that it is customary, all things being equal, to continue medication as prescribed by the regular doctor.

What could be the doctor's motive for murder? He had a lucrative practice and was well respected. Why would he purposely set out to destroy a partially paralyzed elderly woman who had a limited life expectancy? There were those who believed that Dr. Adams set out to make Mrs. Morell totally dependent on him after he realized that she was addicted to drugs. By abruptly increasing her dosage he intended to influence her in any way he wished concerning her will. It must be remembered that Mrs. Morell was an extremely wealthy woman. When her will was finally probated, her estate amounted to £175,000. A tidy sum today, in 1950 this amounted to a fortune.

Detectives uncovered a form, signed by Dr. Adams, which had secured Mrs. Morell's cremation. One of the questions of the form was, "Have you, as far as you are aware, any pecuniary interest in the death of the deceased?" The doctor answered in the negative, although it is quite clear that he was aware he would receive the Rolls and the silver under the terms of Mrs. Morell's will. Mrs. Morell was cremated the day after her death.

It took six years before the doctor was asked his reason for lying on the cremation form. His only explanation was that he had not lied from any sinister intent, but only to circumvent red tape and get on with the cremation.

On the day of Dr. Adams' arrest he made a statement that was to haunt him throughout his trial. In response to being advised of his rights he told a Scotland Yard detective, "Murder? Can you prove it was murder?" Not exactly the utterance of an innocent man.

During the Adams trial it was revealed that Mrs. Morell was not in pain while under the doctor's care.

Expert medical opinion stated that morphine and heroin should be used only if the patient is suffering agonizing pain. Mrs. Morell was irritable and had trouble sleeping. Other drugs should have been used, and furthermore, Dr. Adams, as a competent physician, would know this. In fact, two expert medical witnesses swore that the dosages prescribed by Dr. Adams were certain to cause death.

Dr. Adams' defence attorneys produced experts of their own, who stated that it is impossible to tell exactly how an 81-year-old partially paralyzed woman died. Remember, Mrs. Morell's body had been cremated, so it was impossible to perform an autopsy. The defence doctors claimed that it is quite common for an individual who has suffered one stroke to suffer a second, fatal one. In fact, this was suggested to the jury as an alternative to murder. This theory was ridiculed by the prosecution and contributed the only levity to an otherwise grim affair. Crown attorneys likened this second stroke theory to the instance of a man walking on a railroad track and being struck by a train. Is it reasonable to assume he had a heart attack a moment before the train struck, and therefore death was not due to a train accident but to a heart attack?

The crux of the Adams' trial revolved around the definition of murder. Murder is an act in which the intent is to kill, and that does in fact kill. A doctor attending a dying patient is compelled to take those measures necessary to relieve pain and suffering, and if his efforts incidentally shorten life, that is not murder. If he deliberately and knowingly cuts off life, that is murder. In the Adams case it was totally irrelevant if life was shortened by a day or by a year. If the intent to kill was there, it was murder. If a doctor errs in his judgment, and institutes measures that effectively terminate life, that is not murder. Intent was of the essence in the Adams case.

Despite the suspicious circumstances surrounding Dr. Adams and his particular brand of medicine, he received the benefit of reasonable doubt. The jury took only 44 minutes to find him not guilty.

The trial of Dr. Adams for Mrs. Morell's murder stands alone, and I have tried to relate the salient points of the tedious trial as fairly as possible. However, the reader should know that, at the time, Dr. Adams came under strong suspicion for the deaths of two other patients. In fact, at the preliminary hearing that preceded the Morell trial, it was alleged that Adams murdered two other rich patients, a Mr. and Mrs. Hullett. While Adams was in custody, the bodies of these two suspected victims were exhumed, but as the Crown took no action against Adams in this regard, we can only assume nothing incriminating was found.

After his acquittal of the murder of Mrs. Morell, Dr. Adams was arrested and charged with sixteen counts of forging medical prescriptions and contravention of the Cremation and Dangerous Drugs Acts. He pleaded guilty to fifteen of these charges and was fined £2,400.

As a result of these disclosures, the General Medical Council of England had Dr. Adams' name struck off the Register of Medical Practitioners. John Bodkin Adams never practised medicine in England again.

DR. BOB RUTLEDGE
1951

Gentlemen who monkey around with other gentlemen's wives sometimes find themselves in all sorts of hot water. Occasionally the hot water becomes positively scalding.

It takes two to tango, but it takes three to triangle. Let's follow the three corners of our love triangle to the day all hell broke loose.

Bob Rutledge Jr. was born and raised in Houston, Texas. He always found schoolwork relatively easy, and from the very early grades he was considered college material. He breezed through high school and entered university as a pre-med student. While still an undergraduate Bob had a strange but pleasant experience.

In 1943, Bob met a U.S.O. singer, whose group was entertaining soldiers at Fort Des Moines. He married the girl. Four hours later she left town with her group. I can find no record of what the young couple did during their short four-hour marriage, and maybe it is just as well. Bob and his blushing bride were divorced two years later without ever seeing each other again.

Bob went on to graduate as a full-fledged medical doctor. He then joined the navy and served 15 months at a navy hospital in Boston. It was during his stint in the navy that he met Sydney. I should explain—Sydney was a girl, and quite a girl at that. She had long blonde hair, and a very well proportioned figure spread over a height of six feet. At 23, Syd was a looker. In 1946, Bob and Syd were married. A short time later Bob entered Children's Hospital in St. Louis to specialize in pediatrics, drawing down a cool $25 per week.

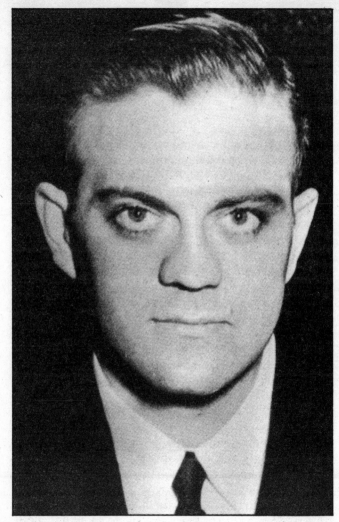

Dr. Bob Rutledge

Syd, who was the daughter of a physician, was well aware of the long training period required to become a specialist. To pass the time and supplement their income, she obtained a job at the Emerson Co. as a mathematician. Working directly across from her desk was the third member of our triangle, Byron Hattman. Byron glanced up from his drafting table and took in all six feet of the voluptuous Syd.

Byron was a graduate engineer, having received his diploma from the University of Pittsburgh. After a spell in the Marines, he had joined Emerson in St. Louis as an airplane instrument designer. Now 29 years old, Byron was a bachelor without a care in the world. He drove a big car, owned a sailboat, and loved to carry a substantial wad in his pocket.

Day after day Byron looked at the statuesque doctor's wife. In July the Emerson Co. had an outing, a cruise on the Mississippi River. As usual Dr. Rutledge was working at the hospital. Syd went on the cruise with a group of girls from work. For the first time, Hattman struck up a conversation. Soon the pair were enthusiastically discussing sailing. One thing led to another. Hattman invited Syd and some other girls to go sailing the following Saturday. Everyone accepted the invitation.

That weekend the girls had a great time on the boat. The next Saturday was another story. This time Hattman invited Syd to join him alone. Syd accepted and even told her husband of her innocent date. He approved.

The sailing session lasted until 6 p.m. During the trip Hattman impetuously told Syd that he didn't think it could be much fun being the neglected wife of a doctor. That afternoon Hattman made a date with Syd to have dinner. When Syd went home to change, she neglected to tell her husband about the dinner engagement.

We will never know for certain what took place that evening. It all depends on whom you choose to believe.

Sydney was to forever state that she was viciously raped. Hattman always claimed she gave of herself willingly. Whatever happened that night, Syd did not mention a word of the evening's activities to her husband.

Poor Dr. Rutledge found out about his wife's having intercourse with another man in a most disturbing way. He overheard Hattman bragging about his conquest of Syd at another Emerson party—this time a day of golf at the Norwood Hills Country Club. Dr. Rutledge had the day off and decided to join his wife at the company function. Hattman didn't notice him changing his shoes when he was telling a group of employees of his romp in the hay with Syd.

This startling bit of information stuck in the doctor's craw for several weeks. Then he did something about it. He called Hattman on the phone, informing him that he knew what had happened. He issued a warning to Hattman to stay away from his wife. In passing, he also mentioned that it was quite possible Syd was pregnant. The doctor suggested that Hattman cough up $250 for the necessary abortion. Hattman replied tersely that he didn't much care if Syd was pregnant or not. He suggested that the doctor contact his lawyer for anything further. Some weeks later Hattman was advised that Syd wasn't pregnant after all. Nature had merely played one of her cruel little jokes.

Meanwhile Dr. Rutledge and his wife had a tête a tête concerning Hattman. It was then that Syd told him that Hattman had forced himself upon her. He decided to stick by his wife.

During the month of October and the remainder of that fall, the Emerson Co. subcontracted a large job to Collins Radio Co. in Cedar Rapids. Hattman was directly involved in this job and had to split his time between St. Louis and Cedar Rapids. Each Monday he would travel the 300 miles to Cedar Rapids, and check into the

Roosevelt Hotel, where he stayed for two or three days.

On December 15, 1948 he never made the return trip. That morning a chambermaid, with the apt name of Carrie Chambers, found Byron Hattman dead on the floor of Room 729. Beside his head was a large bloodstain and an empty wallet. The room showed signs of a vicious struggle. Bloodstains covered all four walls. The victim had bruises about his face, broken ribs, and assorted cuts about the head. Later the coroner was to state that Hattman had been stabbed repeatedly in the chest. One of the thrusts had punctured his heart, causing death.

Hotel guest Eugene Pastock stated that he had heard a fight at about 5:45 p.m. the previous evening. He assumed it was a domestic squabble and never gave it another thought. Police, knowing nothing of the victim's private life, felt that Hattman had surprised a prowler.

Detectives called at the Collins factory where Hattman worked. Kenneth L. Ebershoff told them that Hattman had confided in him that he was having trouble with a Dr. Rutledge, because of the doctor's wife. Officials of the Emerson Co. also informed the police that Hattman didn't have an enemy in the world, except for a Dr. Rutledge, whose wife seemed to be having an affair with Hattman.

The police, now hearing the name Rutledge from two independent sources, decided to probe a little deeper into the activities of the good doctor. When they found out he had spent Monday night at the Montrose Hotel in Cedar Rapids, he became a prime suspect. Just as quickly Rutledge appeared to have an airtight alibi.

On the day of the murder, Tuesday, Dr. Rutledge had checked out of the Montrose early in the morning. The office manager of a garage, Mrs. Bee Nichols, stated that the doctor had brought his car into her garage that same morning to have a water pump repaired. He picked the car up before noon. Rutledge had been short of cash and told Mrs. Nichols he would send her the money through the mail. At 7:30 that evening Mrs. Nichols received a long distance call from Dr. Rutledge, apparently from St. Louis, confirming that he had just dropped her cheque in the mail. If this were so, he couldn't be the killer. It had been established that the murder had taken place in Cedar Rapids at 5:45 p.m. There was no way Dr. Rutledge could travel the 300 miles to St. Louis in one hour and forty five minutes.

Cedar Rapids detectives weren't taken in by the flimsy alibi. They filled the tank of their car with gas and took off for St. Louis. When the tank neared empty, about one hour and 45 minutes out of Cedar Rapids, they began canvassing gas stations. Sure enough, the police found the station where the doctor had not only purchased gas, but had made the long distance call to Mrs. Nichols, leading her to believe that he was calling from St. Louis.

When detectives went to pick up Dr. Rutledge, the ever faithful Sydney asked them to wait. The doctor was in the bathroom. During those few minutes Rutledge administered poison to himself and collapsed on the way to the police station. He survived, but while being washed in the hospital it was revealed that he had used large quantities of pancake makeup to hide the many superficial scratches he had obtained during his fierce struggle with Hattman.

The Rutledge murder trial was a sensation. The doctor and his wife held hands throughout the trial. Long queues formed each morning to catch the juicy details of the seduction of the doctor's wife. Much was made of the fact that Sydney could have left her job at Emerson at any time to escape Hattman's advances. She left the day his body was found in the hotel room.

Dr. Rutledge was found guilty and received a sentence of 70 years in prison. After serving only a year, he appealed and was released on $40,000 bail pending the results of his appeal. The Rutledges moved to Houston, Texas, where the doctor opened a clinic for the treatment of children.

On April 4, 1951, an Iowa court ruled that the doctor had received a fair trial. The next day Dr. Rutledge bought a long plastic hose. He drove his car to an isolated road about 15 miles from Houston where he attached the hose to his exhaust pipe and placed the other end inside the car. He then closed all the windows and turned on the gas. A drilling contractor found his body at 5:30 that evening.

In 1952, a court decision was made as to who would receive the proceeds of Dr. Rutledge's $10,000 insurance policy. While in the navy he had named his first wife of four hours as the beneficiary, and had neglected to change it after his marriage to Sydney. A judge decided to divide the $10,000. Ironically, Rutledge's wife of four hours received the bulk of the money.

DR. FLORENCE WHITTINGHAM
1953

This is a love story with an unhappy ending.

It all began in Dunedin, New Zealand, when Dr. John Saunders met Dr. Florence Whittingham. John was the resident medical officer at Dunedin Public Hospital. At 27 years of age, the handsome young medic could look forward to a long and fulfilling career. The nurses at the hospital considered him to be a prize catch.

When Florence, who was the same age as John, arrived at the hospital, the two doctors were in contact with each other on a daily basis. Florence was the hospital's new house surgeon.

It didn't take John long to become infatuated with his new surgeon. The doctors dated. Florence fell in love. In a matter of weeks, John and Florence were inseparable. Around the hospital they were considered a pair who would eventually marry.

John wrote to his mother in Christchurch that he had met and was going steady with an attractive surgeon, whom he would one day bring home for a visit. Mrs. Saunders read a lot into her son's letter. Although she knew John had often dated, this was the first time he had ever mentioned bringing home a girl to meet his mother.

In May 1953, John proposed to Florence. She was thrilled. Theirs would be the ideal marriage. Everything was stacked in their favor. They had similar cultural backgrounds, were the same age and both were totally committed to their medical specialties.

In the weeks following their engagement, they were only separated on those occasions when their medical duties kept them apart. When Florence informed John that she was pregnant, he was ecstatic. He pointed out that because of the pregnancy they should get married as soon as possible.

The happy couple travelled to Christchurch to visit with John's mother. Mrs. Saunders was almost as excited as her son at the news of his impending marriage to pleasant, attractive Florence. Right up until John told her Florence was expecting his baby.

That's when Mrs. Saunders changed her tune. Was John sure he wasn't marrying because of the baby? Up to that time, John had not even thought that he was being coerced into marriage. After all, he loved Florence. Her pregnancy had been nothing less than a thrilling and happy circumstance. John's mother even suggested that if they really and truly didn't want to marry, she would adopt the baby.

John and Florence left Christchurch in a state of shock. Their happy news was now muddled. A doubt had been placed in John's mind.

Back at the hospital, the two doctors worked together, but there was a subtle change in their relationship. John was no longer the warm, concerned lover. It appeared to Florence that he no longer wanted their child. When she faced him with this accusation, he reproached her for thinking irrationally, but Florence didn't believe he was telling the truth. In July, she procured an abortion. When John was informed of the abortion, he appeared to be relieved. As the weeks went by, he started to ignore Florence. In time, their relationship, which could have lasted a lifetime, was over. In September, John officially called off their engagement.

Florence was devastated. Of necessity, she and John had to work together at the hospital. There were many days when Florence dragged herself to the hospital, performed surgery and dragged herself home. Life was not worth living without John. His reaction to escaping being a husband and father was one of total relief. Soon he was dating other women, in particular nurse Frances Kearney.

News of John's dating came to Florence's attention. It was not easy to take. Only months earlier she had been pregnant with John's baby. They had been planning a life together. Now she had nothing.

Dr. Florence Whittingham purchased a .303 rifle and a box of ammunition. The weapon lay in her room for some weeks, untouched. Maybe she would one day put the fear of God in John's mind. Maybe that would bring him to his senses. On the other hand, it was possible that she would never use the rifle.

The decision was made for her when she heard that John was taking Frances Kearney to a hospital party to be held at Dr. Brian McMahon's apartment. A few days before the party, which was scheduled for December 12, Florence phoned Frances and said, "This is the mother of John Saunders' child speaking."

Frances was astounded, but recognized Florence's voice. She asked if this was Dr. Whittingham. There was a pause and then a sobbing yes. Frances hung up and immediately informed John of the irrational phone call. He suggested they ignore it. That was a mistake.

John took Frances to the party. Florence took along her trusty .303, concealed under her coat. She arrived late and sought out John. Most of those attending the affair were in one room. Suddenly a shot emanating from the hall brought the merrymaking to a sudden halt. The shot was followed by a bloodcurdling scream.

The partygoers ran out to the hall. There was Dr. John Saunders on his knees, blood pouring down his shirt. Florence was at his side, babbling to the dying man, "Listen to me John!" But John Saunders was beyond listening. Slowly, he slumped dead to the floor. As he did so, Florence dropped beside him. When she was lifted from his fallen form, a .303 rifle was evident beside his body. Florence screamed, "John's dead! He's dead!" Everyone there knew that.

Dr. Florence Whittingham was taken into custody and charged with murder. Her sensational trial commenced on February 8, 1955. The entire story of love and death was recounted in detail. The prosecution claimed that it was purely and simply a case of premeditated murder. Florence had purchased the weapon, which she had carried to the party with the express purpose of killing John Saunders.

Florence's defence was based on her statement that she had taken the rifle to the party in order to frighten John, not to kill him. The trial lasted six days, after which the jury retired to reach their verdict. They deliberated 12 hours before returning a verdict of guilty, not of murder, but of manslaughter, with a strong recommendation to mercy. In reaching their verdict, they stated that they felt the rifle had discharged accidentally.

Dr. Florence Whittingham was sentenced to the light term of three years imprisonment.

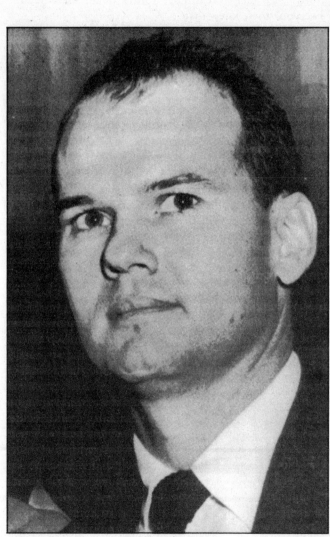

Dr. Sam Sheppard

DR. SAM SHEPPARD
1954

Mayor Spencer Houk looked at the clock beside his bed, yawned, turned over and went back to sleep. The mayor had every right to be at peace with the world. It was going to be a beautiful summer's day in his town, Bay Ridges, a fashionable suburb of Cleveland.

It was 5:30 a.m., July 4, 1954. The phone on the mayor's night table rang. From that moment, nothing was ever quite the same in Bay Ridges. Dr. Sam Sheppard, who lived only a few houses down West Lake Rd., was on the other end of the line. He urged the mayor to come to his house immediately. The doctor sounded frantic. He said, "For God's sake, Spen, get over quick! I think they've killed Marilyn!"

Houk and his wife dashed over to the Sheppard residence. They found Dr. Sam sitting in his den, barechested. His trousers were wet and he was wearing a pair of loafers. He mumbled, "They killed Marilyn."

Mrs. Houk proceeded to the second floor. She peered into the Sheppards' bedroom and was shocked to see Marilyn Sheppard's body on the twin bed closest to the door. Mrs. Houk, a strong woman under the circumstances, felt for a pulse, but there was none. She went downstairs, told her husband what she had seen and called police.

From Sam Sheppard and other witnesses, police reconstructed the evening preceding the murder. Sam and Marilyn had visited with neighbors, the Aherns, earlier in the evening. After having cocktails, the Aherns and their children, together with the Sheppards, returned to the doctor's residence, where they had dinner. After dinner, they listened to a ballgame on the radio and watched T.V. Dr. Sam curled up on a couch and dozed off. Around 12:30, the Aherns left. The next thing anyone knew of events at the Sheppard residence was when Mayor Houk received the phone call from Sam.

When police questioned Sam that morning, it was noted that he had a bad bruise around one eye and complained of pain in his neck. His two brothers, Stephen and Richard, both doctors, whisked their brother to Bay View Hospital.

Back at the house, authorities examined the body and the premises. The bedroom was spattered with blood. Marilyn was lying on her back, with the upper portion of her body exposed. Her head was a mass of blood and the bed clothing was soaked. Later that same morning, Mayor Houk's son found a bag in some bushes leading to the beach while he was searching the grounds around the Sheppard home. Inside the bag were Sam Sheppard's wristwatch, a pocket chain and a ring.

Dr. Sheppard told his story. He claimed that Marilyn retired for the night and went upstairs alone. Someone was there in hiding. When Marilyn screamed, he raced upstairs and in the darkness received a blow to the head. Down he went, stunned, if not unconscious. Regaining his senses, he heard movement downstairs. He raced after his attacker and overtook him on the beach. Once again, he was struck down and rendered unconscious. Sometime later he regained consciousness and staggered inside the house. He made his way upstairs, observed his wife, and called his friend, Spencer Houk.

Dr. Sam's story seemed reasonable enough, but a strange thing happened in Cleveland. A mood swept over the city. Rumors spread that the neurosurgeon had orchestrated his wife's death and because of his wealth and influence, he would get away with murder. Evidence pointing to guilt was highlighted in the press, while evidence pointing to his innocence was overlooked.

Dr. Sheppard was taken into custody and charged with his wife's murder. On October 18, 1954, he stood trial. Because his brothers had tended to his wounds, they testified as to the seriousness of his injuries. Sam's claim that he had been twice knocked out in the course of two battles with his wife's killer was in the main substantiated by Sam's brothers. Such testimony was felt to be biased. Sam wore a neckbrace during the entire trial. Cleveland papers called it trickery.

An expert insinuated that the murder weapon may have been a medical instrument, the inference being that the doctor would have easy access to such an instrument. Maybe the most damaging evidence to Sam's cause was the appearance of his mistress, Susan Hayes. She testified that she had been intimate with Sam for over two years. Their most recent tryst had taken place only a month before the murder. No array of character witnesses swearing Sam was a loving, caring husband could overcome sexy Susan.

And so it went — no absolute proof, but a strong insinuation of guilt. In summing up, the prosecuting attorney left the jury with several questions. Why was Sam, a big, well-conditioned athlete, so easily knocked out? Why had he not turned on the light switch when he went upstairs to answer his wife's call for help? Why didn't he phone the police from his wife's bedroom? Why did he chase the prowler who had just slain his wife and overpowered him? If he had to chase the murderer, why didn't he pick up a weapon when several were handy?

The questions boomed across the courtroom and had a great effect on the jury, although upon close examination not one actually connected Dr. Sam to the murder. Sam Sheppard was convicted of murder in the second degree and sentenced to life imprisonment.

When prison gates closed behind the doctor, his brothers began a campaign to gain a second trial. Meanwhile, Dr. Sam stayed active in his own way.

For some reason, certain women are enamored of men convicted of murder. Ariane Tebbenjohanns, a glamorous, wealthy German divorcee, corresponded with Sam in prison. Eventually she flew over from Dusseldorf to meet her pen pal. The unlikely pair were soon married.

Steven and Richard Sheppard retained famed lawyer F. Lee Bailey to act on their brother's behalf. He succeeded in obtaining a new trial for his client based on the grounds that "prejudicial publicity" had deprived Dr. Sam of a fair trial 12 years earlier.

At his second trial for the murder of his wife, Dr. Sam was found not guilty. He was free at last, but life held little happiness. It took over a year to have his medical licence reinstated. Once again practising medicine, he soon was faced with so many negligence suits that insurance companies refused to provide him with coverage.

The love story with the German beauty came to an end. Ariane obtained a divorce. She claimed that Sam had threatened her with a knife.

Dr. Sam had always been a bodybuilding enthusiast. He turned to wrestling to support himself. A broken and lonely man, he married the 19-year-old daughter of a wrestling friend. Six months later, his health began to deteriorate. His young wife implored him to consult a doctor, but Sam refused.

On April 6, 1970, Dr. Sam Sheppard died of natural causes.

DR. YVES EVENOU
1955

Simone Deschamps was a 43-year-old seamstress when she met Dr. Yves Evenou. It was an innocent enough meeting. Simone called on the doctor for a medical. Five years later, the seamstress and the doctor would provide all of France with one of the juiciest trials that country has ever enjoyed.

Simone wasn't beautiful, nor did she have a voluptuous figure. But beneath the seamstress' plain appearance beat the heart of a passionate, love-starved woman who had never fulfilled those urges we all possess in various degrees. Dr. Yves Evenou would change all that.

On the surface, Evenou was a kind and gentle doctor with a fine reputation. Tucked away at home there dwelt his ever loving wife, Marie-Claire, and 12-year-old daughter, Francoise. They had no idea the good doctor was leading a double life. When not in his office or at home, Evenou was seldom without a glass of port in his hand. He loved the ladies and indulged in every perversion known to man with various ladies of the night. Sometimes, the doctor invented unique perversions of his own. Let's face it, he was one wild and crazy guy.

In Simone he met a lady who was easily led. After a few dates, she was not only in love with the medic, but totally under his influence. No perversion was too weird for Simone. Always half sloshed on port, Evenou didn't treat Simone with a great deal of respect. He would often insult her in front of waiters. Despite the humiliations, Simone was madly in love with him and did exactly as she was told.

Probably her most demeaning moments came when Evenou brought home strangers to have intercourse with her while he watched. On other occasions, he would urge her to take off portions of her clothing in public places to satisfy some unfathomable personal sexual desire.

The relationship between the odd couple grew stronger. Simone moved into the apartment building where Evenou lived with his wife and daughter. She occupied an apartment on the first floor. What could be more convenient? The doctor slipped down the stairs at every opportunity to indulge his peculiar sexual urges. Simone never disappointed. For five years the unholy alliance flourished.

Something had to give. It all happened within a period of 24 hours one day in 1955. Dr. Evenou was slugging back his port with Simone at one of their regular watering holes, Madame Porree's Restaurant on Avenue des Allies. He brought up the subject of murdering his wife. The dear woman was ill, which would make the task that much easier. Evenou is reported to have said to Simone, "We can't go on unless she is removed. You must remove her. You have taken her place. You have a duty to me."

Simone, after years of obedience, listened wide-eyed. She agreed. It seemed the logical thing to do. The doctor went on, "Marie-Claire must die today. You must kill her. I will make preparations, of course. I shall see that everything is made ready. I think it would be as well if you stabbed her. Yes, that would be best."

Simone excused herself. Evenou ordered some more port. Twenty minutes later, Simone returned to the restaurant. She smiled as she showed her lover the menacing hunting knife with the horn handle which she had just purchased. Evenou approvingly took the weapon in his hand. It was perfect.

Together, the tipsy doctor and the dressmaker left the restaurant. Evenou told Simone that they must kill his wife that very night. He briefed her on his plan and told her to wait in her apartment. The waiting was the hard part. Simone admitted later that although she was nervous, she never once thought of not going through with the plot to kill Marie-Claire Evenou.

A few floors up, in his own apartment, Evenou enjoyed the last dinner his wife would ever prepare. Although she was ill, Marie-Claire insisted on cooking her husband's meals. After eating, the doctor went for a short walk around the neighborhood. No doubt he felt that he had created the perfect sex partner to share in his perversions. This would be the ultimate perversion. He had trained Simone to such a degree that she would kill for him on command.

Evenou returned to his apartment and called Simone. He said only one word, "Now." Simone had prepared herself as her lover had instructed. She wore only high-heeled red shoes and black gloves. She slipped her overcoat over her nude body and carefully placed the horn handled knife into a pocket. One last touch. Simone applied bright red lipstick as Evenou had suggested. She was ready. She walked up the stairs leading to her lover's apartment, making certain that she wasn't seen by anyone.

Evenou was waiting. He removed the knife from Simone's pocket and placed her coat over a chair. He assured her that everything had been arranged. He had taken the precaution of giving his wife a sleeping pill earlier on. The doctor led Simone to his wife's room. Gently, he pulled down the bedclothes. Then he pointed to his wife's body and told Simone, "Look. There is the heart. Now strike there."

As always, Simone obeyed. Nude except for her black gloves and red shoes, she struck. Maybe her mind was willing, but she hesitated. The knife came down, but it was a slow, sluggish blow which hardly broke the skin.

Marie-Claire awoke with a start. "Yves, Yves!" she cried as she looked up at her husband's smiling face.

The consoling husband responded, "I'm here, you were having a nightmare." Marie-Claire rose to get out of bed. Her husband clutched her in his arms and shouted to Simone to strike. Simone slashed out with the hunting knife. All hesitation had left her. She swung wildly time and time again. In all, she inflicted 11 stab wounds. Finally, Marie-Claire lay still in death.

In a daze, Simone returned to her apartment. She washed her blood-smeared body before turning to the incriminating knife and gloves. They too were dripping blood. Simone washed them carefully and then took needle and thread and sewed them into her mattress.

Dr. Evenou called police, but his story of an intruder didn't stand up under close scrutiny. His love affair with the lady in the ground floor apartment was discovered by police. It didn't take long for Evenou and Simone to confess to the murder, each accusing the other of being the mastermind behind the killing.

Arrested and lodged in prison, awaiting trial, Dr. Evenou took seriously ill. His years of drowning himself in port, coupled with his dissipated lifestyle, had taken its toll. The good doctor died, leaving Simone alone to face the music. And face the music she did, to the fascination of the entire country.

Eighteen months after the crime was committed, Simone, now 48, stood trial for murder. The woman who sewed dresses for a living, who up to five years earlier had led a humdrum existence, stood in real danger of being executed. On the advice of her counsel, Simone revealed her every thought and action from the time she had first met the evil doctor.

The details were so explicit and perverse that the judge often cleared the courtroom before allowing Simone to continue. Her defence rested on the influence the doctor wielded over her. She was depicted as nothing more than a tool in the hands of an evil man who had used her to kill an unwanted wife.

The prosecution demanded Simone's head. They claimed that cunning alone had enabled her to sew the gloves and knife into her mattress.

Simone was found guilty, but displayed great remorse for what she had done. It was this remorse which provided the court with the necessary "extenuating circumstances" required to reduce the sentence from the guillotine to life imprisonment.

And that's how it all ended for the seamstress who, six years earlier, had called on a doctor for a routine medical.

DR. PETER DRINKWATER
1959

Dr. Peter Drinkwater seemed to have the world by the tail when he completed his medical training at St. Bartholomew's Hospital in London, England in 1959. Within a year, he married and, together with his wife Christine, set out to conquer the world. The doctor joined the Royal Army Medical Corps. For five years he served in Germany and later in British Guyana. Then something went wrong.

During the latter years of his term in the army the handsome young doctor deteriorated rapidly. He drank with a vengeance, mixing his drinks with drinamyl and amphetamines. After he attempted suicide by placing a pistol to his head and threatening to pull the trigger, he was returned to England and discharged.

Dr. Drinkwater joined an existing medical practice in Reading, where he continued his wild lifestyle. He had been fined several times for reckless driving when he struck and killed an elderly cyclist. The man was dragged 40 yards before the doctor stopped his vehicle and ascertained that the cyclist was dead. Dr. Drinkwater then drove away, neglecting to report the accident until 30 minutes later. After this latest brush with the law, his driver's licence was suspended for three years.

It was during this time that the doctor began to pay a great deal of attention to one of his patients, blonde, shapely Carole Califano. Carole lived in apparent harmony with her hubby, Gerrard, until Peter Drinkwater came upon the scene. Gerrard owned a chain of hairdressing salons, which provided him and his wife with more than an adequate living. As time passed, the doctor evidently provided Carole with more earthy pleasures. Whatever the reason, Carole became infatuated with Drinkwater and Drinkwater became infatuated with Carole.

In May 1971, Christine Drinkwater divorced her husband on the grounds of cruelty. Seems the good doctor habitually came home loaded to the gills with booze and drugs. He liked to beat up Christine just for fun. She took their two children with her when she left.

Three months later, Carole Califano left her husband and eight-year-old daughter, Bridgetta. She moved in with Dr. Drinkwater. In the months preceding the move, Carole had been taking drugs given to her by her lover. Those who knew her well claimed that she was now under the complete domination of Peter Drinkwater.

For about a year, Carole was something of a zombie in the doctor's hands. Her continued use of drugs often threw her into a state of depression. On July 2, 1972, Dr. Drinkwater frantically called another medic, Dr. King, and implored him to rush over to his home in Hemsby, Norfolk. Drinkwater said it was an emergency, and sure enough it was. Carole was lying face down on her bed. She was dead.

Peter Drinkwater told the first detective at the scene that Carole had been extremely depressed because he had been in contact with his wife. She believed that he was about to break up their relationship, which was not the case. Obviously distressed, she had decided to end it all with an overdose of drugs. The investigator bought that one for the time being. An autopsy indicated that Carole had died as the result of four substances taken in combination.

Once again, Dr. Drinkwater was interviewed. This time he told a different story. He and Carole had argued about her suspicion he was returning to his wife. He grew exasperated and filled a syringe with a fatal dose of drugs.

Then he told her to go ahead if she wanted to end it all. Naturally, he stressed that he never dreamed she would actually carry out her suicide threat. Now he was racked with guilt.

There matters would have stood forever had police not decided to search the Drinkwater bungalow. They uncovered Polaroid photographs of Carole alone and with Peter in pornographic poses. An English court was later to describe them as "lewd and bizarre."

For the third time, the doctor was questioned. He gave yet another version of the events leading up to his mistress' death. He admitted that he had injected the fatal drugs, but had done so at Carole's request. Dr. Drinkwater explained that Carole had asked him to render her unconscious so that he might take the pornographic poses. She had often made the same request and he had complied with her wishes.

It was quite a story, but it wasn't believed. Dr. Peter Drinkwater was taken into custody and charged with Carole Califano's murder. In December 1972, he stood trial for murder at St. Albans.

The doctor was the star of the show. From the witness stand, he explained that he and Carole had had normal sex relations right up until a month before Carole's demise. In fact, they had intended to get married when both were free to do so. Drinkwater had even given Carole a wedding ring as proof of his honorable intentions.

Despite this gesture, Carole grew despondent, mainly over her inability to gain custody of her daughter, who had been sent to Italy to live with one of her husband's relatives.

To ease the tension of the relationship, Drinkwater purchased a Polaroid camera, not to take obscene pictures of Carole, but to have some pure, clean fun. A couple of weeks after he purchased the camera, Carole suggested they take some erotic photos.

They decided to get high before embarking on their photographic adventure. He injected Carole with pentathol, while he downed amphetamine tablets to get in the mood. Drinkwater testified that he had become so high he was incapable of working the simple camera mechanism. Carole, who had been rendered unconscious was disappointed next morning when he told her the photographs had not been taken.

That same day, the doctor attended to his medical practice fortified by pills. Surprisingly, his practice did not suffer, nor did his patients ever realize that on most days he was under the influence of alcohol, drugs, or both. With office hours concluded, the doctor downed a couple of gin and tonics at a nearby pub and picked up a bottle of wine to take home.

He and Carole were sharing the wine when, according to Drinkwater, she suggested they continue the erotic picture session of the previous night. He went on to state that Carole said the picture session would serve to cement their relationship. She also suggested that he use pentathol to put her under. He removed Carole's clothing and carried her into the bedroom where he gave her another injection to ensure that she would be asleep when he posed her body.

Next morning, Dr. Drinkwater woke up to find Carole lying face down in bed beside him. He assumed she was asleep. After getting up to make tea, his head cleared. He ran to her side and took her pulse. Carole was dead. In a futile effort to revive her, he injected a respiratory drug directly into her heart.

Dr. Drinkwater then told the court how he sobbed at the bedside of his only true love. He emphasized that at no time did he intend to murder Carole. He only intended to comply with her wishes to take erotic photographs.

The doctor went on to say that he panicked and made up the suicide story. He placed the body exactly as he found it, tidied up the scene, and called Dr. King. He believed Carole must have suffocated during the night. Above all, he wanted to keep the pornographic photos and erotic activities of the night before from investigators.

Prosecution attorneys painted Dr. Drinkwater as a cold-blooded killer, who lied at the least provocation. The defence asserted that at no time did he intend to kill Carole.

In the end, the jury was asked to delve into the doctor's drug-hazed mind. Did he intend to murder Carole? It would still be murder if death ensued from an action on his part which he knew might cause physical harm. On the other hand, if there was no intent to kill or physically harm the victim, but merely to put her to sleep, the correct verdict would be manslaughter.

After close to six hours deliberation the benevolent English jury found Dr. Peter Drinkwater innocent of murder but guilty of manslaughter. He was sentenced to 12 years imprisonment.

DR. BERNARD FINCH
1960

Dr. Bernard Finch had everything any man could ever want. He had a big home, lovely wife, two children, a Swedish maid, a Cadillac, and a thriving practice. He also had a mistress.

In August 1956, an 18-year-old girl named Carole Tregoff was sent to the West Covina Medical Centre in West Covina, California to apply for a position as a receptionist. Carole was a tall, shapely redhead, in full bloom, so to speak.

Doctor Bernie took his time and it wasn't until the winter of 1957 that a cute little apartment was found and rented in the name of Mr. & Mrs. George Evans. Now, for well over a year Bernie and Carole "teamed up" pretty well every day at lunch, and sometimes before work in the morning. Carole had one embarrassing hurdle to get over. You see, she too was married. Her husband, Jimmy Pappa, was not aware of his wife's affair. Their marriage was on the rocks and he and Carole were living together without sharing the connubial couch. It seems Jimmy was the only one who wasn't aware of the torrid romance.

Certainly Barbara Finch knew that something was wrong. She also knew that if she let her husband have a divorce, she would become, under California law, legally entitled to only 50 per cent of his assets. If she could prove adultery, she would get a much larger settlement. Not one to let sleeping dogs lie, Barbara called Jimmy Pappa and told him about his wife. When Carole came home from work that day, Jimmy did the manly thing. He punched her in the mouth. Carole packed up her belongings, left the house and filed for divorce all in the same day.

Meanwhile back at the Finch residence, conditions became intolerable. In May 1959, the Finches were quarreling and fighting on a regular basis. On May 16, Bernie beat up Barbara. On May 20, Barbara filed for a divorce. On May 21, she sought a restraining order that forbade her husband to harm her. At the same time the order prevented him from using or disposing of any funds or property, and as of June 11 the restraining order was signed into the record. At this time Bernie was worth three quarters of a million dollars. Not only could he not touch a penny without Barbara's consent, but every cent of income went into their joint account.

This was the tense state of affairs that existed on the night of July 18, 1959 when Barbara Finch drove up the driveway of her West Covina home. Barbara had taken to carrying a .38 calibre revolver for protection. As she started to get out of her car, she saw her husband and Carole Tregoff walking toward her out of the shadows. Instinctively she reached for her gun and pointed it at the advancing pair. Bernie grabbed the gun and took it away from his wife. He then proceeded to attack Barbara. Her screams were heard by their Swedish maid, Marie Anne Lidholm, who came running to Mrs. Finch's aid. Dr. Finch was in an uncontrollable rage. He grabbed the woman and threw her against the garage wall with such force that an impression of her head was implanted in the stucco wall. Bernie fired a wild shot into the air, and then ordered Marie Anne and his wife into the car. Barbara, fearing for her life, went in one side of the car and out the other, and kept on going. Bernie took off after her. Marie Anne saw her chance and ran to the house to call the police. Later she was to testify that she was dialling the police number when she heard a shot. Bernie admitted firing the gun. He claimed that he was flinging the gun

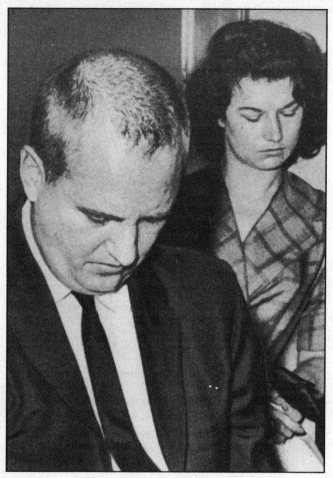

Dr. Bernard Finch and Carole Tregoff

away when his finger caught on the trigger, accidentally discharging the weapon. Firing so haphazardly he proved to be a fantastic shot. The .38 calibre slug made its way through Barbara's back and into her heart.

All this time Carole was hiding in the bushes just out of sight of the action. Only after the police came and finished their investigation did Carole finally get away. She didn't know that Bernie had left or that Barbara was dead. The only living person the police found at the scene was Marie Anne, who had called them in the first place.

Next day, Dr. Finch was arrested and charged with murder. Later Carole was charged as well. At the trial the prosecution brought out the fact that Bernie and Carole had hired an assassin to do away with Mrs. Finch. His name was John Patrick Coady, and he fingered the accused pair from the witness stand. In fact, he received a total of $1,200 for the job that he had no intention of doing. He told a convincing story.

Over and above Coady's damaging evidence, the police had come up with an attache case at the scene of the crime. The case did not contain what your average kindly old doctor would call the essentials. Instead it held two 10-foot-long ropes, an eight-inch butcher knife, a bottle of Seconal, a hammer, a flashlight and a box of .38 calibre cartridges. The attache case was quickly dubbed the "murder kit" by the press.

It took three trials to get a jury to agree, but finally on March 27, 1961, Dr. Bernard Finch and Carole Tregoff were convicted of murder in the second degree. Both were sentenced to life imprisonment.

In 1969 Carole was paroled, and is now employed under an assumed name as a medical records clerk in a hospital in California. Dr. Finch was eventually paroled, and is again practising medicine.

DR. GEZA DE KAPLANY
1962

Dr. Geza de Kaplany had interned at Milwaukee General Hospital in 1957. Later he specialized in anesthesiology at Harvard University, after which he taught at Yale University for a year. In 1961, he was chief medical resident at San Francisco's Franklin Hospital. Still later he accepted the post of staff anesthesiologist at Doctors' Hospital in San Jose, California.

At the age of 36 you might say Dr. de Kaplany was a high achiever. Even in the field of matrimony he hit the jackpot. In July of 1962 he married Hajna Piller, a model and former showgirl. She was gorgeous. Anyone who ever saw Hajna came away impressed by her beauty. Both had immigrated from Hungary to the U.S. while still single.

On the stifling hot night of August 28, 1962, about five weeks after their marriage, Dr. de Kaplany killed his wife. On the day of the crime, Mrs. de Kaplany visited her mother. She arrived home in the early evening and met her husband outside their apartment. They proceeded up to their apartment which was in a two-storey ranch style structure. The young couple commenced to make love on the bed. For no apparent reason Dr. de Kaplany jumped up from the bed. He had an entire torture kit with him. First he beat his wife with his fists. He then tied her hands behind her back with electric cord, and trussed up her feet in the same manner. To stifle her screams he placed tape over her mouth. Dr. de Kaplany slashed at Hajna's breast with a knife. He wasn't through. Calmly donning rubber gloves, he applied nitric acid all over her body.

Despite the fact that the doctor turned the hi-fi on full blast, Hajna's screams pierced the hot summer night, arousing the neighbors' interest. When the police and an ambulance arrived on the scene, they found the doctor pacing outside the apartment in a pair of Bermuda shorts and slippers. Hajna lay nude in agony on the bed, horribly burned over 60 per cent of her body. The officers and medical people had trouble breathing at the scene of the crime due to the nitric acid. Periodically they had to run out of the apartment to get a breath of fresh air.

Hajna lingered in agony for 33 days after the attack before she mercifully passed away on September 30. During the time the doctors struggled to keep her alive she made many statements to the police, but in the end she really could not say just why her husband had done such a terrible thing to her.

On Monday, January 7, 1963, Dr. de Kaplany stood trial for murder. During the trial he changed his plea from not guilty to guilty. Sanity meant the gas chamber, and insanity meant life imprisonment. The trial was a sensation and swayed back and forth on medical evidence attesting to Dr. de Kaplany's mental condition at the time of the murder.

The defence brought forward doctors who claimed he suffered from depression due to leaving an aged mother in Hungary. They said he suffered from paranoid schizophrenia. The prosecution countered with the actual torture paraphernalia which they lugged into court. It made an impressive display in front of the jury—surgical gloves, a quantity of surgical swabs, rolls of adhesive tape, electric cord, one pint of nitric acid, one pint of hydrochloric acid, one pint of sulphuric acid and two knives.

A sensation was caused at the trial when the defence put a young psychiatrist, Dr. A. Russell Lee on the stand. Dr. Lee claimed that de Kaplany suffered from multiple personality. He stated that de Kaplany had two people living in the same body. One was a kind and gentle doctor. The other was brutal and cruel. The brutal one went under the name of Pierre LaRoche. It seems de Kaplany heard some gossip about his wife being unfaithful to him. Instead of dealing with this rumor in a rational manner as de Kaplany would have done, he changed into the aggressive cruel Pierre, and tortured and killed his wife. De Kaplany would change his outward appearance and adopt the personality of Pierre LaRoche, for short periods of time.

Horrible pictures of poor Hajna were introduced as evidence, showing the agony in which she died. The jury could not believe that a man, sane in the legal sense, could perform such atrocities on his wife. They brought in a verdict of guilty. He was sentenced to life imprisonment.

When Dr. de Kaplany was taken away to San Quentin, a reporter asked him one final question as a guard assisted him into the prison van. "Have you any last statement, Doctor?"

"This is the end. I am dead," he replied.

DR. CARLO NIGRISOLI
1964

I am certain that Dr. Carlo Nigrisoli of Bologna, Italy, started out in the practise of medicine convinced that he would uphold every single one of old Hippocrates' tenets. After all, the good doctor came from a long line of distinguished physicians who had practised medicine in Bologna for generations. He had no reason to stray from the straight and narrow.

What went wrong? Iris Azzali, that's what.

Iris strolled into Carlo's clinic one day with a minor ailment. The doctor cured what ailed her, and other things as well. Iris was a willowy, long-legged beauty, with big brown eyes, full seductive lips, and a body that would make the Leaning Tower of Pisa stand up straight and take notice.

From that very first meeting, the older man with a wife and three children at home thought of little else but beautiful, youthful Iris. She, in turn, thought the debonair society doctor so much more intelligent and mature than her regular companions.

How can one put it delicately yet retain a degree of candor? Carlo and Iris met clandestinely at her apartment where their signs of affection soon graduated to physical fulfilment. Oh, what the heck, they hit the sack at every opportunity.

Sure, there were a few anxious moments. Take the time Iris became a tad pregnant. She cried and in general carried on something fierce, but Carlo rose to the occasion. He escorted her to another city, where she obtained an abortion. Presto, her troubles were over.

Now, folks, all this intrigue did not have a good effect on Carlo's wife Ombretta. She realized that Carlo was no longer the loving husband and attentive father he had once been. When Ombretta attempted to discuss her husband's changing attitude toward her, he flew into a rage. Ombretta became nervous and distraught. Something definitely was rotten in the state of Bologna.

The unhappy couple's best friends, Anna and Carlo Frascaroli, soon became aware of the tension between Carlo and Ombretta. Frascaroli, who was also a doctor, had been approached by Carlo, who told him that Ombretta was suffering from nervous exhaustion. Dr. Frascaroli prescribed a series of injections. He began giving the injections himself, but for convenience sake both doctors agreed that Carlo Nigrisoli would continue to give them to Ombretta at their home. Of course, the Frascarolis were totally unaware of Carlo's extracurricular activities with Iris.

Meanwhile, the affair grew warmer. Carlo and Iris couldn't stay away from each other. They took little trips together into the country. Ombretta was miserable. She was losing her husband. The father of her children was no longer interested. On the other hand, Carlo now regarded his wife as an obstacle standing in the way of his happiness with firecracker Iris.

The potentially dangerous triangle exploded on March 14, 1964. It was around midnight when Carlo raced from his bedroom shouting to the servants, "I must get Signora Nigrisoli to the clinic! She has had a heart attack!"

Poor Ombretta was rushed to her husband's clinic, but died without regaining consciousness. Carlo explained, "I had given her a heart stimulant by injection, but it doesn't seem to have succeeded." Carlo was completely distraught, but did muster up enough presence of mind to suggest to the doctors in attendance, "Put on the death certificate that she died from coronary thrombosis." The doctors disagreed with Carlo, feeling that they did not have enough information to be certain of the cause of death.

Suddenly, Carlo extracted a neat little pistol from his inside coat pocket. Raving like a lunatic, he shouted that he would kill himself unless the doctors signed the death certificate. Instead, they calmed him down and called police. In minutes the blubbering Carlo was in a police station answering embarrassing questions. When Italian detectives found out that he had been giving his wife a series of injections, they decided to hold him until the results of the post mortem were revealed.

These results caused a sensation throughout the country. The autopsy showed that Ombretta had died from an injection of curare. Curare is not your average poison, not by a long shot. It's a rare vegetable poison derived from certain South American plants. Some South American Indian tribes treat the tips of their arrows with it for use in warfare. The poison causes paralysis of the muscles, which is quickly followed by an inability to breathe. It has been used medically as a relaxant prior to operations. Dr. Frascaroli stated definitely that he had never used nor prescribed curare for Ombretta's condition.

Dr. Carlo Nigrisoli was charged with his wife's murder. His trial began on October 1, 1964. It was the first trial held in Italy where curare was used as the instrument of death. It was also Italy's first televised murder trial. Adding to the uniqueness of the proceedings, Carlo obtained permission to testify from his cell via a sound system especially set up for that purpose. At no time was he actually in the courtroom, although his voice could be heard and he could hear everything which transpired.

Iris testified, admitting to her affair with the accused man. Dr. Frascaroli related that he had prescribed a nerve tonic for Ombretta to be taken intravenously. Dr. Frascaroli dramatically added that he had instructed Carlo to discontinue the injections a few days before Ombretta died.

It was proven that Carlo continued to give the injections. The prosecution painted the cruel picture of Carlo injecting his wife with curare, which rendered her helpless. He then cleaned up the evidence of his deed and watched as his wife took 20 minutes to die. It was only then that he ran for help.

A well known neurologist, Prof. Domenico, surprised the court when he testified that Ombretta had discovered a hidden bottle of curare in her bathroom on the day before her death. Realizing that her husband might very well be about to murder her, she visited the professor for advice. He told her to go directly to the police, but she wouldn't listen. She insisted on trying every possible method of winning back the affection of her husband. The professor did convince her to take a trip the next day in order to be out of Carlo's reach. The advice came too late. On the day following Ombretta's visit to the professor, she was dead.

On February 14, 1965, the 117-day trial came to an end. Dr. Carlo Nigrisoli was found guilty of murder and sentenced to life imprisonment.

DR. JOHN BRANION
1967

Dr. John Branion Jr. owed a lot to his father. John Sr. was born into deep south Mississippi poverty, with all the ugly ramifications the location and social standing held for members of the black community at the turn of the century.

Despite all odds, John's father made his way north, attended the University of Chicago Law School and became a prominent attorney. He devoted his life to championing the causes of his people. His one son would never know the hard times he had endured.

John Jr., to the chagrin of his parents, was a mediocre student. His marks in school didn't warrant acceptance to any medical school in the U.S. Like many well-off families, the Branions found a medical school in Europe which would accept their son. John applied himself and returned home with his medical degree. He interned in Chicago, specialized in obstetrics and gynecology and set up a practice. Within a very short while, Dr. John Branion was a wealthy, respected physician.

To add to his lustre, John married into a prominent black family when he wed Donna Brown, the daughter of banker Sidney Brown. The influential, socially prominent Branions of Chicago had two children. Theirs was a success story that Hollywood writers would deem too perfect to be accepted by the public.

Surely there had to be a flaw in the perfect couple's life that begged to be uncovered, but such was not the case. Years passed. The Branions accumulated the trappings of wealth. Cars, designer clothing and a classy 10-room apartment were theirs to enjoy. In time, John acquired a substantial stable of racehorses. Oh, sure, there were some whispers of other women, but such whispers are the norm among the wealthy.

Shortly after 11:30 a.m. on December 22, 1967, Theresa Kentra, who lived in the same apartment complex as the Branions at 5054 S. Woodlawn Ave., heard several short reports she thought might have emanated from the Branions' apartment. She paused for a moment, but thought nothing more of the incident.

Accompanied by his four-year-old son, John drove up to his apartment. He told his son to wait in the car while he went inside. John opened the door, walked through the kitchen into a utility room and came across Donna's body lying on the floor. He ran out the back door of the first-floor apartment and called up to Dr. Helen Payne, who lived on the third floor. Dr. Payne and her brother William rushed downstairs. They were met by John, who pointed, "In there. It's Donna."

John hustled his son up to a third-floor apartment occupied by a relative. He returned to his own apartment as William Payne was calling police. In minutes, officers were at the scene. They were greeted by John, who told them, "I haven't touched her. As soon as I observed the lividity in her legs, I knew she was dead." Dr. Payne introduced herself to the officers, explained that she was a medical doctor, advised them that she had examined the body and confirmed that Mrs. Branion was dead. By now John had seated himself, covered his face with his hands and was quietly sobbing.

It was three days before Christmas. It seemed natural to suspect that some gun-happy thug had robbery in mind when he had entered the Branions' home. People have been murdered before for a few gaily wrapped Christmas presents under a tree. When homicide detectives arrived, they immediately checked for evidence of forced entry, but found none. The officers searched the house with John. Nothing was missing. They theorized that Donna Branion must have opened the door to her killer, whom she no doubt knew.

Crime lab technicians examined an electric iron cord they found beside the body. It appeared that Donna's killer had attempted to strangle her. When she put up a fierce struggle for her life, he started shooting. Four cartridge cases were found under the body.

An autopsy indicated that Donna had been shot seven times. Three of the bullets had gone through her hands as she raised them in a futile effort to ward off her attacker. Any of the other four bullets could have caused her death.

Dr. Branion was questioned by detectives. He told them that he left his office at 11:30 a.m. to pick up his four-year-old son, which took only five minutes. He then drove to East Fifty-Third St. to pick up Maxine Brown for lunch. Maxine, a relative of his wife's, couldn't make lunch because of an unexpected business appointment. John drove home and discovered his wife's body. He went on to tell investigators that upon entering his apartment he called out to his wife. When he didn't get a response, he felt something wasn't right. He told his son to wait in the hall while he continued on into the kitchen. When he turned on the light of the utility room, he was shocked to find his wife's body on the floor. John noticed the lividity present in her legs and realized she was dead. That's when he made his way outdoors and called Dr. Payne.

That was the doctor's story. It was concise and straightforward. A couple of things caught the attention of the detectives. There were a number of guns in the apartment's laundry room. When asked about the weapons, John told the investigators that he was a gun collector and owned about 25 guns. He kept his collection in the laundry room. John checked out the guns for the officers and assured them that none was missing, nor had any of the guns been recently fired.

The first day of the investigation into the tragic death of Donna Branion was fast drawing to a close. Detectives left the Branion residence. The next day, two days before Christmas, would bring further attempts to find out who had murdered the socially prominent doctor's wife. No doubt investigating officers would be interviewing Dr. Branion in the morning.

Surprise! Next day homicide detectives learned that early that morning John, his 13-year-old daughter and four-year-old son had taken off for a skiing vacation in Vail, Colorado.

Folks, that's not a natural reaction to suddenly losing a wife. No question about it, Dr. John Branion had managed to gain the full attention of the police.

Now that the doctor had managed to draw suspicion to himself, investigators delved into his lifestyle, checked out his friends and rechecked his statement. They learned that Theresa Kentra, who lived in the Branions' apartment building, heard several loud reports on the day of the murder a few minutes after 11:30 a.m. About 20 minutes later, she heard the doctor shouting to Dr. Helen Payne for assistance.

Joyce Kelly, a teacher at John's son's nursery school, stated that she had seen Dr. Branion enter the school between 11:45 and 11:50 a.m. and help his son on with his coat. This was in conflict with John's original statement to police in which he had said that his son had been waiting outside when he came to pick him up.

Tracing the doctor's every move on the day of the murder, detectives next drove to the office of Maxine Brown, who had been unable to keep her luncheon date with the doctor. Although she knew John well, that was the first time he had ever asked her out for lunch. Investigators felt that the good doctor had planned on having Maxine with him when he came across his wife's body. He had no way of knowing that an unexpected business appointment would make it impossible for Maxine to lunch with him and his son.

John had claimed that he had known immediately that his wife was dead because of the presence of lividity in her legs. Dr. Helen Payne told police this was impossible. She had examined Donna's body moments after John had found it and there had been no lividity evident at that time.

Little by little, John's statements were found to contain small discrepancies. Firearm experts reported that Donna had been killed with a Walther PPK pistol, the same type made famous by James Bond in the movies. An examination of John's guns turned up no such weapon. He swore he had never owned such a weapon. Detectives pressed on. They learned that the doctor had a girlfriend, his nurse, Shirley Hudson. She had accompanied him on his skiing trip to Vail. That little caper, detectives all agreed, takes a certain type of man. After all, Donna's body was being prepared for a post mortem while John, his mistress and the kiddies were off skiing in Colorado. Folks, in better circles, that is rarely done.

Dr. Branion was a busy little gynecologist. He had another lady on the line, Anicetra Souza, who admitted to being a good friend, but swore there was nothing of an intimate nature between her and John.

When detectives learned that John had asked his wife for a divorce and had been refused, they were sure they were on the right track. Now they set out to prove that Dr. Branion had had sufficient time to commit the murder by retracing his every move, starting at his office at Ida Mae Scott Hospital. They drove to his home, allowed time for the shooting, drove to Branion's son's nursery school, proceeded to Maxine Brown's office and then back to Branion's apartment. Investigators traced the route a half dozen times. Each time they gave the benefit of the doubt to the doctor. On every trip, they proved that he had plenty of time to commit the murder and show up at the times stated by various witnesses.

Although officers knew they had a strong circumstantial case, they desperately wanted to locate the murder weapon. Once again they searched the Branions' laundry room, which was more of a workshop, looking for any clue that would lead them to the Walther PPK. Sure enough, in the doctor's work bench, they found a box which had contained a new Walther. Since John had sworn he had never owned such a weapon, detectives had every reason to believe they had the right man.

Inside the box was a paper listing the serial number of the pistol and on the outside of the box the name of the importer, Joseph Galeff and Sons, New York City. They had sold the gun to Bell's Gun Shop in a Chicago suburb, where it had been purchased three months earlier by James Hooks, a good friend of none other than Dr. John Branion.

Hooks initially denied any knowledge of the weapon, but when he was shown a copy of the gun shop's invoice with his name on it, he admitted that he had bought the gun. He went on to tell the officers that he had given the gun to John Branion as a birthday present.

That was it. John was picked up at his office and charged with his wife's murder. An Illinois jury took only seven hours to find him guilty. The presiding judge sentenced him to not less that 20 years or more than 30 years imprisonment.

John appealed his conviction and, in an unusual move, was granted bail until his appeal could be heard. Bail was set at $5,000, which meant that only a $500 payment was required for him to gain his freedom. No question about it, strings were pulled to spring the murderous medic. The public was outraged, but despite the outcry, John walked.

Branion's next legal ploy came in the form of a petition

for permission to move to Cheyenne, Wyoming. Once again, an exception was made and John was allowed to relocate. He packed up bag, baggage and nurse Shirley Hudson and headed west. Once there, he married Shirley. Then, in a whirlwind matrimonial merry-go-round he divorced Shirley and married Anicetra Souza. Remember her? She was the girlfriend who claimed her relationship with John had never been an intimate one. John wasn't through. He divorced Anicetra, remarried Shirley, divorced Shirley and remarried Anicetra. That comes to four marriages and three divorces in the two-year period he was appealing his conviction for murdering his first wife.

Finally, John's conviction was affirmed by the Illinois Supreme Court. He immediately flew the coop, forfeiting his bond and was charged with unlawful flight to avoid incarceration. Over the next few years, he kept one step ahead of the law.

In 1972, John was spotted in Khartoum in the Sudan. Now on Interpol's hot sheet, he was next traced to Uganda, where he worked for the Department of Health and later became personal physician to dictator Idi Amin.

When the mad dictator's reign collapsed, John fled and remained at large until Interpol learned that he was in Kuala Lampur, Malaysia. Once more, he managed to stay one step ahead of the law. He fled back to Uganda, but evidently that country had had enough of the evasive doctor. In 1983, Ugandan authorities advised the U.S. that they had their man under lock and key.

Chicago detectives flew to Entebbe and brought back the fugitive. On November 2, 1983, after a 12-year chase, John was back in a Chicago courtroom. From there he was transported to the Illinois State Prison, where he served seven years. His sentence was commuted on August 7, 1990, when a tumor was discovered on his brain.

A month later, 64-year-old Dr. John Branion died in the University of Illinois Hospital.

DR. JOHN HILL
1969

When blonde and beautiful Joan Robinson met John
Hill, there were those who said that the young couple
were made for each other. On the surface it appeared that
way.

Joan was the only daughter of multi-millionaire oil
man Ash Robinson. Ash had eyes for only two things in
this world — money, and his daughter Joan. As a result
she had her every desire fulfilled from the day she was
born.

John Hill was brought up in a small southern Texas
town, but had a bright future ahead of him as a plastic
surgeon when he met Joan in 1957 in Houston. Within
15 years of their first meeting both would die violently.

Although Joan and John appeared to be happily married, it wasn't long before the deep-rooted differences in
their backgrounds and interests rose to the surface. Joan,
who at 27 had gone through two unsuccessful marriages,
had a consuming interest in horses. From the age of five,
when she first learned to ride, horses were to play a major
role in her life. By the time she met John she was one of
the leading horsewomen in the U.S.

John took no interest in his wife's equine pursuits.
Other than his lucrative medical practice, he had an
obsessive love of classical music. The doctor played several instruments, including the piano, at a near professional
degree of excellence.

Later Ash Robinson would present his daughter and
son-in-law with a beautiful new home. John went about
indulging himself in the real passion of his life, music. He

remodeled and equipped a ballroom-sized area of his home into a music room.

In 1960 the Hills had a son, Robert. This normally thrilling event only served to interrupt Joan's appearances at horse shows for a short while. Soon servants were tending to Robert. John apparently cared little for his new son, and continued building up his medical practice, while spending more and more time in his elaborate music room. Ash Robinson adored Robert and spent every moment he could with his grandson.

In August 1968 Joan and John visited a summer camp to pick up their son Robert. While there John met Ann Kurth, an attractive divorced mother of three sons, who was visiting her boys at the same camp. John became madly infatuated with Ann. The successful doctor pursued Ann with notes, flowers, and other expressions of undying love, until Ann began to appreciate the attentions paid to her by John Hill. Soon she was in love with the dashing, attentive doctor. When Ann broached the subject of Joan, she was assured that the Hill marriage was on the rocks and that John would soon obtain a divorce.

Quite out of character, John impetuously moved out of his home, leaving Joan only a brief note of explanation, and moved in with Ann. When John served Joan with divorce papers, Ash Robinson was furious. No one was going to treat his little girl in such a shoddy manner. Ash met his son-in-law and threatened him with ruin if he didn't reach a reconciliation with Joan. Ash had provided John with cars, a mansion, indulged his musical taste to the fullest, and assisted him in building up his medical practice. Influential Ash Robinson would see to it that the house of cards came tumbling down if John didn't return to his wife. The meeting between the two men resulted in John signing an agreement stating that he was sorry that he had acted irrationally and that he would give up everything Ash Robinson had provided if he did not return to the side of the everloving Joan.

John moved back with Joan.

In the light of future developments, the evening of March 9, 1969 holds a great deal of significance in the lives of Joan and John Hill. On that night the Hills were entertaining when John's telephone pager went off. He was called away and did not return until after 11 p.m. Upon his return he offered the guests pastries which he had brought with him. He insisted that his wife eat the one particular pastry which he set before her. Evenings later John was again interrupted while his wife was entertaining guests. Again he returned with pastries and insisted that his wife eat one in particular.

Within 48 hours Joan became dreadfully sick. John prescribed bed rest. Two days later Joan developed a raging fever. Frantically her maid called John to come home to tend to his wife. John arrived home and made arrangements for his wife's admittance to a small hospital. Eyebrows were raised when the desperately ill woman wasn't sent to the Texas Medical Center located less than 15 minutes from the Hill residence. Dr. Hill kept insisting his wife would be fine, and that her illness was of a minor nature. In the wee hours of the following morning, Joan Hill died in agony.

Ash Robinson took his daughter's sudden death very hard. It was incomprehensible to him that a healthy young woman could die so suddenly with her husband, a well known doctor, being readily available at all times.

Dr. John seemed to take Joan's death in stride. He continued his affair with Ann Kurth. Ash Robinson was convinced that his son-in-law had murdered Joan. He approached the district attorney with his suspicions, but was put off.

Less than three months after Joan's death, John married Ann Kurth. The marriage reinforced Ash Robinson's belief that John had killed Joan. Private investigations carried out by Ash Robinson uncovered the strange circumstances of the pastries being served by John to Joan and her friends.

Finally the D.A. impanelled a grand jury, but they failed to indict. Rumors were flying around Houston, when eight months after his marriage to Ann Kurth, John filed for divorce. When the divorce became final Ann Kurth went to the D.A. and talked of her marriage to John Hill. As a result of these revelations the grand jury was impanelled once again. This time one of the leading prosecution witnesses was none other than Ann Kurth. Miss Kurth stated that John had confessed to her that he had made up a horrible poison of human excrement and administered it to Joan, causing her sudden and fatal illness. She also told of her former husband's strange Jekyll and Hyde personality when, on two occasions, he turned on her with a syringe.

Dr. Hill was charged with the crime of murder by neglect. His trial commenced in March 1971. It was now two years since Joan Hill's death. Dr. Hill, who apparently didn't let any grass grow under his feet, now had another lady friend. Connie Loesby had one thing Joan and Ann didn't have. She had a genuine interest in music. John wanted to marry her, but heeded his lawyer's advice to wait until the conclusion of his trial.

Hill's trial proved to be one of the most sensational ever held in Houston. Ann Kurth was the acknowledged star of the piece. Wives are not allowed to testify against their husbands. However, as Ann was no longer married to John, she was allowed to testify, providing she limited her testimony to events which occurred before she legally became Mrs. John Hill.

Ann became emotional while giving testimony, and blurted out that John had told her in detail how he had killed Joan. This was inadmissible evidence and the judge ordered a mistrial.

Soon after the mistrial John married Connie Loesby and tried to begin a new life. It wasn't easy. The doctor's practice had quite naturally suffered but as the months went by the notorious Hill case was put on the back burner. That is, until one fateful day in September 1972.

The Hills had just arrived home by plane from a trip to the west coast. While John paid off the cabby, Connie walked to the front door of their home. Connie rang the doorbell and was shocked to be greeted by a man wearing a green Halloween mask. The stranger grabbed Connie by the neck, dragging her into the house. He said only, "This is a robbery."

By this time John was at his wife's side. As he grappled with the intruder Connie managed to break free and run towards a neighbor's home. While running she heard gunfire.

Police were on the scene in a matter of minutes. Dr. Hill had been shot in the shoulder, chest and right arm. His killer had grotesquely placed tape over his mouth, eyes and nose. The doctor's second trial for murder was scheduled to take place in two months, but someone had taken justice into his own hands.

Houston police were successful in tracing a young hood named Bobby Vandiver, who confessed that he, together with prostitute Marcia Mckittrick, had killed Dr. Hill. According to Vandiver he had accepted the contract killing from Lilla Paulis, a shady but influential acquaintance of Ash Robinson.

Vandiver and Mckittrick told all, but before Lilla Paulis came to trail, Vandiver was killed while attempting to escape from jail. Mckittrick turned state's evidence and revealed all the details of the killing. As a result Lilla Paulis was found guilty and sent to prison for life. To this day she has not verified that Ash Robinson was involved in the contract killing. Robinson has never been charged with any crime.

DR. CLAUDIUS GIESICK
1973

Intricate murder plots, disguised to look like accidents, oftimes go asunder. Occasionally, relatives smell a rat and assist police.

Stanley and Josephine Albanowski of Trenton, New Jersey, simply couldn't believe that their beautiful daughter, Patricia, had been a hit-and-run victim in New Orleans. They hired a lawyer, who contacted New Orleans police. The lawyer's inquiry was routinely turned over to Det. John Dillman, who responded by getting in touch with Patricia's mother.

Mrs. Albanowski informed the policeman that Patricia had moved from New Jersey to Dallas in November 1972. About two weeks before Christmas, her daughter met Dr. Claudius Giesick, who swept Patricia off her feet. Patricia had never received such attention from a man in her life.

Handsome, debonair Giesick showered gifts and attention on naive Patricia. As a token of his affection, he gave her a pair of St. Bernard puppies. On January 2, 1973, they were married. Dr. Giesick reportedly gave his wife a new Monte Carlo automobile for a wedding present. The happy couple took off for Miami, where they were to board a cruise ship for a trip throughout the Caribbean. Patricia was on Cloud 9.

Then, disaster struck. At first, the Albanowskis thought it was a minor setback. Their daughter phoned them from her motel room in New Orleans. She was alone in her room when she informed them that her car was in a repair shop. She had just walked some distance

214

to pick up a pizza.

Nine hours later, Patricia's parents were told that their daughter was dead, the victim of a hit-and-run driver. Dr. Giesick was understandably beside himself with grief.

The doctor explained to investigating officers that he and his wife had gone for a midnight stroll. They were walking back to their car when Patricia and he raced across the street. They didn't see the vehicle approaching. Early next morning, Patricia died in hospital without regaining consciousness.

A few days later, the Albanowskis met their son-in-law for the first time at their daughter's funeral in New Jersey. The doctor was accompanied by a man who was introduced to them as his spiritual adviser, Rev. Sam Corey.

A couple of things bothered Josephine Albanowski. A few hours before the tragedy, Patricia had told her that her car was in a garage for repairs, yet the doctor said they were returning to their car when the hit-and-run took place. Why the discrepancy in stories? Mrs. Albanowski informed police that the doctor's first wife had also been a hit-and-run victim. On the phone, Patricia had mentioned that her life had been insured by her husband.

Det. Dillman did some poking around. He found out that Dr. Giesick had picked up the Monte Carlo from the repair shop eight hours before the death of his wife. Dillman looked up the officer who had taken the hit and run report. The officer had been sympathetic to the doctor, which was only natural. The poor man had just lost his wife on his honeymoon.

When the officer had asked where Dr. Giesick's own vehicle was, the doctor had pointed to an Olds Cutlass parked in the motel parking lot. The officer took the doctor's word and didn't bother to check. There didn't seem to be any point. Now Dillman wondered if the doctor had an ulterior motive in pointing to a motel patron's car.

It was also revealed that Dr. Giesick had paid his bill at the Ramada Inn with a credit card issued to Dr. Charles Guilliam. The motel's management assured the detective that this is often done. They merely checked to insure that the credit card was good.

More inquiries uncovered the fact that Dr. Giesick had taken out a $50,000 life insurance policy with Farmers Insurance Group of Houston, Texas. The policy had a double indemnity clause, doubling its value in case of Patricia's accidental death. It had been purchased five days after the wedding.

Dr. Giesick had attempted to collect on this policy the day after Patricia's fatal accident, but had been delayed until the insurance company completed their investigation. Later, Dillman would learn of another insurance policy, issued by Mutual of Omaha for $200,000 on Patricia's life.

Det. Dillman was now sure that Patricia Giesick had not met with an accident. He found out that Giesick lived in Dallas, but could not reach him on the telephone. Without benefit of interviewing his chief suspect, Dillman delved into the history of the dead girl and her husband. He learned that Patricia had worked for a couple of days in a body massage parlor. Naive Patricia didn't know the place was really one of several such parlors, which were fronts for a prostitution ring run by Rev. Sam Corey. It was Reverend Sam who officiated at Patricia's wedding and later accompanied her husband to her funeral in New Jersey.

You couldn't miss Reverend Sam. He weighed more than 350 pounds and stood no more than five feet nine inches. Among those who knew the Reverend Sam's real vocation, he was called the Massage Parlor King.

While the net of circumstantial evidence was slowly encircling Dr. Claudius Giesick, he was picked up for passing a bad cheque in Dallas. By the time Dillman arrived in Dallas to question his man, Giesick had been released on bail posted by Rev. Sam Corey.

Det. Dillman interviewed Rev. Corey, who admitted knowing Dr. Giesick for some time. He had had dinner with the Giesicks a few days before they left on their honeymoon. He claimed he had learned of the tragedy from Patricia's mother, who had phoned him while Patricia was unconscious in hospital. Dr. Giesick had called him a few hours later, advising him that his wife had died. He invited the doctor to stay at his house in Dallas. Giesick accepted his invitation and together they had flown to Trenton, N.J. for the funeral.

Dillman had no trouble checking Corey's story. The Albanowskis swore they had not called Corey and stated that the first time they had seen him was at their daughter's funeral.

Dillman proceeded to learn the address of Dr. Charles Guilliam, whose credit card had been used by Giesick to pay his bill upon checking out of the Ramada Inn after his wife's death. Mrs. Guilliam informed the detective that her husband was not at home. She appeared nervous. When asked about Giesick, she told the investigator that he was a business associate of her husband's.

While interrogating Mrs. Guilliam, Dillman noticed the two Guilliam children playing with a pair of St. Bernard puppies in the backyard. He well remembered that Giesick had given Patricia a pair of St. Bernards. Dillman was sure that Dr. Guilliam and Dr. Giesick were one and the same man.

Finally, Dr. Giesick was interviewed and confirmed that he had picked up the Monte Carlo hours before the accident. The vehicle was examined by police. Near the left front tire, technicians removed two hairs which matched hairs removed from Patricia's head.

There seemed little doubt that the scheming doctor, who lived two lives, one as Dr. Guilliam, a family man with two children and the other as Dr. Giesick, had, together with a con artist minister, orchestrated the hit and run death of an innocent girl from out of town. The motive, a whopping $300,000.

Dr. Giesick and Rev. Corey were picked up and charged with murder. Giesick made a deal in exchange for being allowed to plead guilty to manslaughter.

Dr. Giesick revealed the entire plot. He and Rev. Sam Corey hand-picked Patricia Albanowski. When Patricia found out what was expected of her in the massage parlor, she threatened to quit. The doctor swept her off her feet. On the night of her death, he conned her into taking a walk. Unknown to her, the Rev. Sam Corey was waiting for the pair to appear. He roared down the road with his car lights extinguished. Dr. Giesick tripped Patricia, sending her sprawling into the path of the car.

It took the jury only 20 minutes to find Rev. Sam Corey guilty of first-degree murder. He is now serving a life sentence in Louisiana State Penitentiary.

Claudius James Giesick was sentenced to 21 years imprisonment. On May 17, 1986, after serving 11 years in prison, he was released from custody.

Katherine (Guilliam) Giesick was not charged with any crime.

Det. John Dillman is no longer with the New Orleans Police Dept. A book, Unholy Matrimony, later made into a TV movie, describes in detail how the persistent work of a dedicated police officer brought two heinous criminals to justice.

DR. CHARLES FRIEDGOOD
1976

To all outward appearances Dr. Charles Friedgood had the world by the tail. A successful surgeon, he owned a large eighteen-room home in the affluent Kensington section of Long Island's North Shore. He was the father of a grown, well educated family, and above all was the husband of Sophie, his loving wife of 28 years.

It just wasn't that way at all. Dr. Friedgood, who was in his mid-50s, neglected his wife. He arrived home late for meals, sometimes by hours. No matter what the occasion Sophie never started a meal without him. She waited, and when he finally arrived, she argued, she screamed, and she bickered. To make matters more frustrating, Friedgood ignored his wife's outbursts, and never offered any excuses for his tardiness.

In 1967 Friedgood became infatuated with his Danish nurse, Harriet Larson. Although Harriet wasn't a beauty, she was attractive. Initially the doctor kept his relationship with Harriet a secret, but soon he was carrying on an open affair. For years his daughters, Toba, Esther, Beth, and Debbie had believed that Harriet was nothing more than a faithful employee. Gradually the truth became known to them. Typically, Sophie was the last member of the family to accept the fact that her husband was keeping another woman.

All semblance of secrecy crumbled when Harriet became pregnant. Early in 1972 she flew to Denmark, where she gave birth to a boy, who was named Heinrich after Dr. Friedgood's dead father. When she came back to the U.S., Friedgood set Harriet and Heinrich up in an

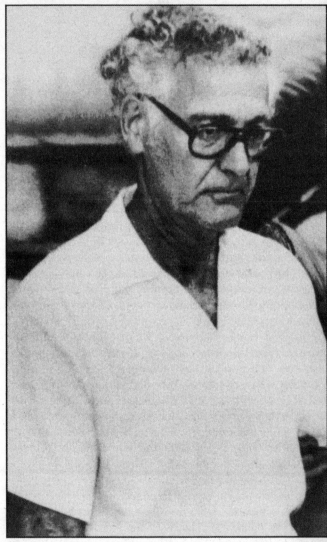

Dr. Charles Friedgood

apartment not far from his home. He paid her an allowance of $1,000 a month. Two years later Harriet found herself pregnant once more. Again she returned to her native country. This time she gave birth to a girl, Matte, with Friedgood at her side. He had told his wife that he was attending a medical convention in Arizona, when in reality he flew to Denmark.

When Harriet and the two children returned to the U.S., Friedgood obtained a larger apartment for his second family, again quite close to his home in Kensington. He helped furnish it with older pieces from his own home that Sophie had discarded. Friedgood was under pressure from Harriet to obtain a divorce from Sophie. He convinced his mistress that because of financial difficulties incurred while he was purchasing a hotel, he had signed over everything he owned to Sophie, almost a million dollars in stocks, bonds, and cash. As soon as the deal cleared the courts, he would be free to marry, but in the meantime Sophie legally owned everything.

At the same time the doctor tried to explain away Harriet to his wife by telling her that he couldn't dismiss his nurse because she had been witness to several documents he had signed concerning the same financial deal.

As the Friedgood girls grew up they came to know and like their father's nurse. Sometimes they were puzzled when little Heinrich would hug their father and call him Papa. Later they realized that the child was named after their own grandfather, and that besides, he bore a striking resemblance to one of their brothers. One by one the Friedgood girls married. Each of their husbands eventually learned of the strange, rather open relationship their father-in-law had with his nurse. Occasionally one of his daughters would approach her father and beg him to explain his relationship with Harriet. Friedgood wouldn't hear of such scandalous talk. He assured them that it was nothing more than that of doctor-nurse. He was so convincing that sometimes his children believed him.

Naturally, Sophie, who over the years had been humiliated by her husband literally hundreds of times, fought back in the only way she knew. She screamed at him, "Go to your whore!", "Sneak away to your bitch!" Friedgood had the exasperating habit of calmly reading his newspaper during these tirades.

The tense relationship between Charles and Sophie Friedgood could not continue indefinitely. Things came to a head on June 17, 1975. That evening Charles and Sophie had a date to meet for dinner at Lundys Restaurant in Brooklyn. Sophie was in good spirits, having heard that Harriet was in Denmark. She arrived promptly at 6 p.m. Typically, Friedgood was late. Sophie sipped wine as she waited for him for over an hour.

After dinner, at approximately 8 p.m., the couple drove in separate cars to their accountant's home, where they were expected. They arrived at 8:30, stayed one hour, and then drove home. At 11 p.m. Esther called her parents from New Jersey. It was an exciting time for her. She and her husband had both just received their law degrees. Esther had a good chat with her mother and father. Moments later Charles and Sophie retired to their bedroom. They were alone in the big house.

We will never know exactly what happened in the Friedgood bedroom after 11 p.m. that night. Later, at Dr. Friedgood's trial, a medical examiner reconstructed the events as they must have unfolded.

Sophie and Charles undressed. Sophie lay in bed while Charles went to a filing cabinet in his study. From the top drawer of the filing cabinet he removed a long needle and syringe. He then filled the syringe with demerol.

Sophie, lying on her back in bed, had no way of knowing she had only moments to live. Charles pounced on his wife, firmly grasping one outstretched arm above her head. As Sophie struggled, Charles injected the demerol up under her armpit. The doctor then held his wife help-less for the ten or twelve minutes it took the demerol to take effect. Sophie screamed frantically. The big house was empty. There was no one to hear.

A few minutes passed. Sophie became drowsy. Her efforts grew weaker. Charles lifted his wife's other arm, and once more jabbed the needle under her armpit. Injections in her thigh and buttocks followed. She lay quiet, but was still breathing. Charles turned his wife's limp form over. He gave her one last injection between the ribs directly into the liver. Sophie stopped breathing.

Dr. Friedgood replaced the needle and syringe in the top drawer of his filing cabinet and returned to his bed-room. He went to sleep beside the lifeless body of the woman who had been his wife for so many years.

Next morning Dr. Friedgood went to work as usual. Lydia Fernandez showed up for work at the Friedgood residence as she did every day. She tidied up around the house, and found it a bit strange that Mrs. Friedgood had not left her a note telling her when she should be awak-ened. Later that day, at 1 p.m., Lydia found Sophie Friedgood dead in her bed.

Dr. Friedgood was notified of his wife's death. He hur-ried home. He told of Esther's call the night before, of going to sleep, of waking up, of Sophie kissing him good-bye. It was shocking. His wife must have had a stroke after he left her. Because Sophie had suffered a stroke years before, it was assumed that she had suffered another one.

In keeping with the Friedgood's religion, steps were quickly taken to have Sophie buried in her hometown of Hazleton, Pennsylvania, the following day. Dr. Friedgood signed his wife's death certificate.

News of Sophie's death spread throughout Kensington. Something clicked in police chief Raymond Sickles' memory. While he didn't know the Friedgoods personally, he recalled that one of the Friedgood daughters had once frantically called him because her mother and father were having a terrible row. When one of his men arrived at the Friedgood residence they found nothing more than the usual family dispute. Sickles learned that Dr. Friedgood had signed his wife's death certificate. Although there was no law preventing a medical doctor from signing a spouse's death certificate, it was unusual. Normally another doctor would have been called upon to sign the certificate.

Sickles decided to inform the Nassau County Police of his suspicions. Officials felt that Dr. Friedgood's actions were so unusual that they consulted Dr. Leslie Lukash, the county medical examiner, who agreed that the funeral should be delayed long enough for an autopsy to be performed. Detective Thomas Palladino was dispatched to Hazleton to see to it that the burial did not take place as scheduled.

While he was mourning at the funeral chapel, Dr. Friedgood was first made aware that the police were concerned about the manner of his wife's death. Under threat that a court order would be obtained granting the autopsy, Dr. Friedgood gave his permission to proceed. He had no choice.

A post mortem was performed at St. Joseph's Hospital, while Detective Palladino looked on. Unbelievably, Dr. Friedgood insisted that he be allowed to observe his own wife's autopsy.

The autopsy revealed that at the time of death Sophie's stomach had been full. How could that be? The meal she had eaten the night before at 8 p.m. would have been digested long before 9 a.m. when the doctor left for work. Sophie must have died within six hours of having eaten the meal. Dr. Friedgood must have been lying when he stated his wife returned his parting kiss the morning after she consumed that meal. She was positively dead at that time.

Dark red bruises were found under the armpits, on the thigh, buttocks, and on the chest. Testing indicated that demerol had been injected in each bruised area. A lethal amount had been injected directly into the liver.

Detectives returned to Long Island hoping to find the needle and syringe in the Friedgood home. While detectives searched the first floor rooms, Dr. Friedgood was able to whisper to Esther, "Upstairs! File cabinet, bottle, syringe — top drawer."

Esther looked in her father's eyes. The surgeon held her stare. A father was to be obeyed and protected. Esther calmly strolled upstairs to her father's study. From the top drawer of the filing cabinet she extracted two bottles and a syringe and placed them in a paper bag. Trembling, she lifted up her dress and put the death kit inside her underpants.

Back downstairs Esther told her sister Toba her terrible secret. After the detectives left she showed her sister the contents of the paper bag. One of the bottles was marked demerol. The Friedgood children discussed their father's plight and his obvious guilt with their husbands that night. Meanwhile, Esther had hidden the syringe and bottles in an upstairs closet. She revealed their location only to her father. The death kit promptly disappeared from its hiding place.

A few days later Dr. Friedgood forged his wife's signature to documents dated prior to Sophie's death, giving him access to several of her safety deposit boxes. He forged authorization to sell several of her securities as well. In all, he gathered up $600,000 in cash, negotiable bonds, and jewelry. He then called his daughter Debbie and told her that his doctor had advised him to get away for a few days. No amount of questioning could get him to reveal his destination. Debbie's husband, realizing that his father-in-law's mistress was in Denmark, was convinced that Friedgood was about to skip. He called the police.

Teams of detectives manned the phones calling Kennedy Airport, canvassing overseas flights. There was no one named Friedgood, or anyone matching Friedgood's description flying to Denmark, but the airport computers did come up with a Friedgood flying to London.

Just as Dr. Friedgood's plane was about to take off, it was instructed to return to the terminal. Friedgood was taken off the plane. A search of his luggage revealed the $600,000 horde. Dr. Friedgood was arrested and charged with the murder of his wife. At his murder trial, his children testified against him. In January 1977 he was found guilty and received the maximum sentence possible — 25 years to life imprisonment.

In 1978 New York State passed a law known as the Dr. Friedgood Bill, making it illegal for doctors to sign death certificates for relatives.

DR. LEWIS GRAHAM
1980

Every major city has at least one infamous domestic murder which becomes indelibly associated with that city. Who can forget the case of Charles Stuart of Boston, who killed his pregnant wife and then staged an attack on himself, or Toronto's Peter Demeter, who orchestrated his wife's murder while he was away from their home?

Shreveport, Louisiana, was the locale of one such crime. The murder took place on March 31, 1980 at 4:12 a.m.

Dr. Lewis Graham and his wife Kathy lived with their three children; David, 16, Eric, 12 and Katie, 8, at 2033 South Kirkwood Dr. in a fashionable section of Shreveport. Lewis had come into an inheritance which gave him an income of $100,000 a year. This was in addition to his substantial salary as a professor of biochemistry and a researcher at the Louisiana State University Medical Centre.

The Grahams were in the process of constructing a custom built home when, in a few short minutes, in the wee hours of a Monday morning, all their lives were to change forever.

Here's what happened according to Dr. Graham. He and his wife went to bed as usual on Sunday night. The children were asleep in their rooms. The first indication that anything was amiss occurred when Lewis thought he heard a scream, which was immediately cut off. At the same time he was thrown from his bed onto the floor. In the pitch blackness, he was picked up, jostled momentarily and thrown against the bedroom wall. He felt a burning sensation in his side.

Lewis fell to the floor, losing consciousness. He didn't know how much time elapsed before he regained consciousness, but when he woke up he turned on the bedroom light. There was Kathy with her head horribly crushed. A quick glance told Lewis that his wife was dead, but to make sure, he touched her body, which was clammy cold. He left the bedroom, locking the door behind him. Lewis claimed that he didn't want his children to see the terrible sight of their mother's body. He proceeded past his children's bedrooms down to the kitchen, where he located a telephone book and called police. He told police his house had been broken into, his wife was dead and he was hurt.

Lewis then called his neighbor, Carolyn Godwin, whose husband happened to be out of town. She called another neighbor, Jerry Siragusa, who rushed over to the Grahams' immediately. The children were awakened and taken across the street to Carolyn Godwin's home. Then the police arrived.

That was the story Dr. Graham told police minutes after he discovered his wife's body. It is substantially the same story he tells today.

Detectives descended on the Graham residence. Right from the outset, this was no ordinary crime. The Grahams had been married for 17 years. Lewis was a highly regarded professional with an IQ of 132. No hint of scandal had ever come close to touching any member of the family.

Immediately after police arrived at the scene, Lewis was taken by ambulance to hospital. He had a superficial knife wound in his side. The cut took only one stitch to close. Back at the Graham residence, police found pry marks at the back door. On the floor was a blood-smeared short-handled sledge hammer and a six-inch long hunting knife. Both items belonged to the family.

Initially it appeared that intruders had entered the

house, picked up Lewis' knife and grabbed a sledge hammer from a closet before making their way upstairs. Kathy, a light sleeper, might have awakened, screamed and been struck a vicious blow with the sledge hammer. When she moved, she was struck again. Lewis, by his own statement, was dragged from the bed, stabbed and thrown across the room.

Lewis attracted suspicion to himself by his demeanor. He never shed a tear at any time over his wife's death. Carolyn Goodwin and Jerry Siragusa confirmed that he had not acted like someone who had just lost his wife. Detectives listened to Lewis' story over and over. It didn't sit well. After regaining consciousness, would a father walk by his children's rooms without looking in on them? After all, they too could have been attacked by the assailant or assailants. Lewis had no explanation for his illogical behavior.

Then there was that superficial wound. How fortunate. The knife blade only pierced the skin. Children who fall off bicycles and cut themselves often suffer worse injuries than the one supposedly inflicted by desperate men who had just killed a woman with a sledge hammer.

Detectives dug into every aspect of the 39-year-old biochemist's life. They discovered that he was in the midst of a prolonged affair with his lab assistant, Judith Carson. Judith was a married woman with two children. She explained to police that she and Lewis had worked together for years. He had told her that he and his wife were having marital difficulties. Apparently, over the years, Kathy's talkative, outgoing nature had gotten on Lewis' nerves. He had the reputation of being a quiet introvert.

Judith and Lewis worked together in the confined area of a laboratory. They never dated at night, nor did they ever spend a weekend together. About every two weeks, they would rent a motel room at noon hour. Police wondered if Lewis' love for Judith Carson was a motive for murder.

The case against Dr. Graham was totally circumstantial and far from airtight, but three months after the murder he was arrested and charged with killing his wife. He was released within an hour after posting a $200,000 bail bond.

On July 21, 1981, Dr. Lewis Graham stood trial for murder in one of the most publicized trials ever to take place in Louisiana. The details of the night Kathy Graham was killed with a sledge hammer were meticulously rehashed. Most damaging to the accused man was the evidence given by Prof. Herbert MacDonell, a criminologist whose specialty was bloodstain pattern analysis. He was the director of the Laboratory of Forensic Science in Corning, N.Y.

MacDonell had examined the T-shirt worn by Graham in bed on the night of the murder. He related to the jury that he had found hundreds of pinpoint blood spots on the back of the T-shirt. The blood was type A, Kathy Graham's blood type. According to the accused man's story of events which had taken place that night, it was literally impossible for him to have gotten those spots on the back of his shirt. MacDonell explained that the spots were entirely compatible with blood being cast off a sledge hammer being held by Graham as he lifted it over his head and struck his wife.

MacDonell also examined blood found on the front of the T-shirt. This blood was type O, Lewis' blood type. The stain formed a straight line of blood, probably made when the accused partially wiped blood from his own knife.

MacDonell's evidence had a profound effect on the jury. They returned a verdict of guilty of second-degree murder. The convicted man heard the judge's devastating words, "It is the judgment of this court, Lewis Graham, that you are hereby sentenced to life imprisonment at hard labor, without benefit of parole, probation or suspension of sentence."

Such are the vagaries of the justice system that the harsh sentence passed down by the judge would later be drastically altered. On February 3, 1988, outgoing governor Edwin Edwards commuted Graham's sentence to 25 years imprisonment. Nearly two years later, he became eligible for parole. On December 9, 1992, Dr. Lewis Graham was granted a parole and was set free after serving 11 years in prison.

DR. KEN TAYLOR
1984

When Dr. Ken Taylor married for the third time, he
would have to be placed in the high-risk category as far as
faithful, long lasting husbands are concerned. The successful dentist, by his own admission, had always been a
ladies' man.

Ken met wife number one when he was a 21-year-old
dental student at Indiana University. He entered a naval
program which provided him with a scholarship for his
entire education. In return, upon graduation, he was
compelled to serve several years in the navy.

When Mrs. Taylor became pregnant, Ken was not
overjoyed. For one thing, he didn't like the responsibility
of another mouth to feed. In addition, a new baby might
curtail his favorite hobby, that of bedding down with anything in skirts. Ken picked a most inopportune time to
leave his wife. It was in June 1974, in her ninth month.

The reason for the separation was a beautiful stewardess. In October, Ken's divorce became final. He married the stewardess in December. Fast worker, our Ken.

The marriage wasn't a successful one. One night, while
wife number two was asleep in bed, Ken attacked her. He
jumped on her and held a chloroform sponge over her
mouth. The poor woman struggled and managed to roll
off the bed, but Ken again pounced on her. Then, as suddenly as the attack had started, it abruptly stopped.

Ken begged for forgiveness. When his wife suggested
he receive professional help, he agreed and placed himself
in the care of a navy psychiatrist. The doctor believed that
Ken was a maniac. He suggested that the police be called

into the case and that the dentist be charged with attempted murder. Mrs. Taylor took the doctor's advice and Ken was charged.

Another navy doctor attributed Ken's action to his mixing alcohol and drugs. He felt that the violent incident was an isolated one. The charge of attempted murder was dropped. Ken received counselling and the Taylors' marriage seemed to get back on the rails.

In 1979, wife number two gave birth to a baby girl. Ken didn't exactly advertise the fact that he still took dope, drank excessively and slept with every dental assistant at the naval base.

In July 1980, Ken finished his navy service. He opened a dental clinic in Brooklyn, which prospered from the beginning. The practice was so lucrative that other dentists and hygienists were hired. One fine day, Teresa Benigno, a gorgeous young thing, applied for a job as a hygienist. Ken took one look at her figure, face and accessories and knew immediately that Teresa was for him. After a few months of his undivided attention, Teresa became Ken's lover.

Back home, wife number two noticed the tell-tale signs — the missed appointments, the lack of attention, the handkerchiefs smeared with lipstick. The marriage disintegrated and finally, in 1983, was dissolved.

On July 10, 1983, Teresa became wife number three. The happy couple honeymooned at a luxury resort in Acapulco. When Teresa's parents travelled to Kennedy Airport to pick up the newlyweds at the conclusion of their honeymoon, there was no sign of Ken or Teresa. Next day, Mr. Benigno called the Mexican resort and was amazed to learn that the Taylors had checked out three days earlier. A call to the American consular agent in Acapulco gleaned the information that Teresa had been seriously hurt and was in hospital. Dr. Taylor was in jail as the chief suspect in his wife's beating.

Within hours, Ken called his wife's family, explaining that robbers had attacked him and Teresa in their luxurious cottage. He had not been badly hurt and had just visited Teresa in hospital. His short stint in jail had been a farce. The Mexican police had insisted on a $500 bribe before releasing him.

Mr. Benigno and another daughter, Celeste, flew to Acapulco. They found Teresa in terrible shape. She had been badly beaten about the head and her throat had been slashed. She spoke to her father and couldn't tell him much about the attack, as she had not seen her assailants. Unfortunately, Mexican authorities had found cocaine in their room. That's why Ken had been taken into custody. Ken told his father-in-law that no charges had been laid against him. Two days later, the honeymooners were back in the United States. Teresa remained in hospital for another week. Slowly, she made a complete recovery.

The months which followed were the happiest of the Taylors' married life. When Teresa informed Ken that there would be an addition to the family, he appeared to be thrilled. Ken was ecstatic at little Philip's birth. But then his urge to play the field took over and once more Ken began leading a double life. There is some evidence that Teresa took to drugs during this time. Certainly the Taylors were willing drug users at private parties. Sometimes Ken admonished Teresa for being spaced out.

On November 12, 1984, Teresa failed to drop off Philip at her mother's on her way to work at Ken's clinic. Mrs. Benigno called Teresa at home, but received no reply. At about 10:30 a.m., Ken called. He told the family that Teresa had a bad drug problem. She had decided to go away by herself for a while to kick the habit. He had driven her to the airport in Newark and was taking baby Philip to his parents in Indiana. He explained that he couldn't care for the baby himself and didn't want to impose on his mother-in-law. He realized they would be worried and was calling from the road. He didn't know where Teresa was staying, but she had told him she'd be back in a few weeks.

The family couldn't help but think of the incident in Acapulco. Was it within the realm of possibility that Dr. Ken Taylor was some kind of maniac? They went over to Teresa's house and found such items as a half-baked cake and her keys. Unusual for a meticulous housekeeper, who never left the house without her keys. The Benignos reported their daughter missing to police. When Ken returned from the round trip to Indiana, he was questioned by the family and repeated the story he had told them on the phone.

Three days later, on November 15, Neil Griesemer was looking for beer cans along the highway at the bottom of Hawk Mountain in Pennsylvania when he spotted a sleeping bag beside the road. He pulled open the bag, exposing the body of a young woman. Mr. Benigno identified the body as that of his daughter, Teresa.

Dr. Ken Taylor was immediately suspected in his wife's murder. He told police of her movements on the night before she disappeared. According to Ken, Teresa had stayed up while he went to bed. He woke up at 4 a.m. Teresa was still up, spaced out on drugs. They had a long talk and she agreed that she had a drug problem. Later that same morning, at around 8 a.m., Teresa told him that she was going away to deal with her problem on her own. She preferred not to tell him where she was going. He drove her to the Newark Airport and never saw or heard from his wife until her body was found.

That was Ken's story, but police didn't believe it for a minute. When they found a bloodstained earring in the Taylors' garage which matched one found on Teresa's body, they were positive they had the right man. Faced with this incriminating evidence, Dr. Taylor broke down and confessed.

He told detectives that on the night in question he had come downstairs to find his wife strung out on drugs. But there was more. As he came down the stairs, he witnessed her sexually abusing their young son. Their eyes met. Teresa dashed into the sewing room, where the family's workout equipment was kept.

Ken placed the baby in a child seat. Teresa suddenly threw a five pound dumbbell at his head, striking him in the shoulder and sending him sprawling to the floor. She leapt on him like a wild animal. He clutched a bar and struck her on the head, at the same time pushing her off. Teresa rushed at him again. He swung the bar, striking her once more on the head. He could remember little else about the attack, but he did recall cleaning the house of blood, placing Teresa's body in the trunk of his car and dumping the body in Pennsylvania.

Dr. Taylor was arrested and charged with his wife's murder. His case was based on self-defence, but the jury didn't believe his story. Even if his story were true, Teresa was unarmed, so he couldn't have struck out in defence of his life.

Ken Taylor was found guilty of murder in the first degree and was sentenced to life imprisonment with no possibility of parole for 30 years. He is presently serving his sentence and has made four unsuccessful escape attempts since his incarceration.

DR. SAMSON DUBRIA
1991

Dr. Samson Dubria was a rising young star at the Lyons Veterans Administration Hospital in Basking Ridge, New Jersey. The easygoing 28-year-old doctor was respected by both patients and staff. For as long as he could remember, he wanted only to be a doctor. While other young men enjoyed taking part in various sports and dating girls, Sam applied himself exclusively to his studies.

When Sam met 20-year-old Jennifer Klapper, all that changed. Sam was smitten. Unfortunately, Jennifer was not enamored with the young medic, although she respected him and appreciated his gentlemanly behavior. For the first time in his life, Sam made a concerted effort to ingratiate himself with a member of the opposite sex. To a degree he succeeded.

Over a period of months, Sam kept in contact with Jennifer. She made it perfectly clear that she already had a boyfriend and had no romantic interest in the doctor. Despite this rebuff, which would have discouraged a less persistent suitor, Sam continued to pursue Jennifer until he attained what at best could be called a platonic friendship with her. On several occasions, Jennifer invited him over to her home, where he met her parents. They too were duly impressed with Dr. Sam Dubria.

When Jennifer told her parents that Sam had suggested they vacation together, they told her to use her own judgment. The two would cross to the west coast, visit Sam's family in Los Angeles and continue on into Mexico. Jennifer liked the idea, but was perfectly blunt with Sam. She told him that she was thrilled with the opportunity to take an adventurous vacation, but wanted his assurance that sex was definitely not a part of the agenda. Sam agreed.

Off the pair travelled. They took in some of Los Angeles' tourist attractions and visited with Sam's parents. The doctor was a perfect gentleman and a delightful travelling companion at all times.

We now know that Sam secretly yearned for Jennifer, not in any platonic manner, but in a strictly sexual way. He wanted to possess her and meant to have her at some juncture on this vacation trip. He was just waiting for the opportune moment to present itself.

It was a steaming hot day in August 1991 when Sam suggested they stop at the All-Star Inn in Carlsbad on their way to the Mexican border. There would be plenty of time for Mexico in the morning. Sam looked at Jennifer in her skin-tight stretch pants and revealing blouse. It was time. He had come prepared. The chloroform was packed away in his luggage.

We will never know how Sam went about rendering Jennifer unconscious with his chloroform. She lay unconscious on the dingy motel room bed, while Sam ravished her in every way imaginable. It is quite possible that he didn't intend to kill Jennifer, but his intentions mattered little to her, for at some time during the orgy her heart stopped beating.

Dr. Sam Dubria fought an inner urge to panic. He attempted to remain calm and to avoid detection at all costs. Quickly, he replaced Jennifer's pants before calling 911 and shouting into the phone, "Come quick! My girlfriend — I think she is dead!"

Paramedics arrived at the motel to find the doctor attempting cardiopulmonary resuscitation on the beautiful young girl on the bed. They rushed her to hospital, where she was pronounced dead on arrival. Sam was exhausted. Those who witnessed his distress had pangs of sympathy for the young man who had obviously fought so desperately to save his companion and had lost the battle.

No one suspected foul play. There were no marks on the body. The first minor mystery arose when a medical attendant who was preparing Jennifer's body for the post mortem noticed that her tight pants had been put on inside out. He mentioned the strange occurrence to his superior.

Dr. Sam returned to New Jersey. His colleagues sympathized with him. The entire affair had been a traumatic experience, but life goes on. Within weeks, he was his old quiet, confident self again.

In California, Dr. Leone Jariwala, who had performed the autopsy, was puzzled. Jennifer Klapper's heart, brain, lungs and all other organs had been perfectly normal at the time of death. Dr. Jariwala couldn't believe that a healthy 20-year-old woman could collapse and die in a hotel room with a physician present without their being some discernible cause of death. She meticulously checked and rechecked all organs which had been removed from the body. Blood samples were sent away for extensive and complicated toxicological testing.

It took two months, but finally Dr. Jariwala's persistence was justified. The tests indicated that Jennifer had been killed by chloroform. No wonder it had taken so much time to get to the truth. Authorities in California had never before encountered a case where chloroform had been used as a murder weapon.

Detectives flew to New Jersey, where they arrested Sam. So confident was the man of medicine that he waived extradition and accompanied the detectives back to California. Once there, he came up with a rather preposterous story. He told investigators that he and Jennifer had driven behind trucks transporting chemicals. The fumes had made him dizzy and no doubt had proved fatal to Jennifer. No one believed that one. When he was told there was evidence that Jennifer had taken part in intercourse immediately before or at the time of death, he quickly responded that their love-making had been consensual. Knowing that Jennifer had attached conditions before taking the trip, no one believed that one either.

In February 1993 Dr. Sam stood trial for Jennifer's murder. His ridiculous story of how Jennifer had come in contact with chloroform was dismissed by the court. Prosecuting attorneys proved that Jennifer had been drugged with a fatal dose of chloroform. The accused was the only one with her at the time and was the only one who could have administered the chloroform. In summing up, the presiding judge touched on the first hint that foul play had taken place. "It doesn't take much imagination. When taking the pants off, they are turned inside out and the sex act is accomplished. The pants are returned in haste and put on inside out."

Dr. Samson Dubria was convicted of murder, rape and administering an anesthetic during the commission of a felony. He was sentenced to life imprisonment, a term he is currently serving.